A Final Arc of Sky

A Final Arc of Sky

A Memoir of Critical Care

Jennifer Culkin

Beacon Press, Boston

Beacon Press
25 Beacon Street
Boston, Massachusetts 02108-2892
www.beacon.org

Beacon Press books
are published under the auspices of
the Unitarian Universalist Association of Congregations.

12 11 10 09   8 7 6 5 4 3 2 1

This book is printed on acid-free paper that meets the uncoated paper
ANSI/NISO specifications for permanence as revised in 1992.

Composition by Wilsted & Taylor Publishing Services

Library of Congress Cataloging-in-Publication Data
Culkin, Jennifer
A final arc of sky : a memoir of critical care / Jennifer Culkin.
p. ; cm.
ISBN-13: 978-0-8070-7285-1 (hardcover : alk. paper)
1. Culkin, Jennifer 2. Intensive care nursing—United States—Biography.
3. Aviation nursing—United States—Biography. I. Title.

RT120.I5.C815 2009
610.73092—dc22
[B]   2008046810

Many names and identifying characteristics of people mentioned
in this work have been changed to protect their identities.

For Kieran and Gabe, my emissaries to the future

For my parents, Frank and Josephine:
May you be waiting for me there
in the light at the end of the tunnel.

For Ben, Erin, Lois, and Steve

For Howard,
and another thirty-four years, right here

Contents

Chapter One

The Shadow We Cast

When I parked my car at ten minutes to nine that summer morning and dragged my helmet, flight bag, food, and laptop up the stairs at the southernmost of our four helicopter bases, the last dregs of predawn coolness still lingered in the air. I was in a good mood. I had just blasted the B-52's *Cosmic Thing* on my car stereo, playing my favorite tracks over and over like a five-year-old for the hour and a half it had taken me to commute to the base from home for a twenty-four-hour shift. The National Weather Service had predicted temperatures in the nineties, but the heat hadn't yet begun to shimmer off the helipad back behind the fire station where we were quartered.

The fire station is tucked into a rural corner of a medium-sized suburban city, next to a county airfield, and the landscape around it was cleared of its native forest a long time ago. It's as open as farmland in Kansas, dotted with Scotch broom, an invasive weed that is nevertheless lush with tiny yellow blooms each May. The sweep of the earth falls away to volcanic mountains in the distance, still snow-covered even in summer, and on my speed walks around the fire station for exercise I'd come to love it, in spite of the landfill that's practically next door. I loved the light and space, the foothill feeling of the land as it runs imperceptibly up toward the mountains.

The day felt pregnant, though—that occupational precognition I've come to trust and dread. It's a feeling with a dart of fatalism in it, a blind, nonnegotiable foreknowledge, and I've learned the hard way that it's pretty accurate. Not 100 percent infallible, but up there. Whenever the feeling comes on me, I think of the animals who head to high ground before a tsunami, whose nervous systems seem to warn them of earthquakes and floods. Rats deserting a sinking ship.

It was also a Friday in high summer, so no shit, Sherlock, of course we'd be busy. We could look forward to office workers ordering margaritas at outside tables in the hot afternoon and driving home wasted in the dusk. Guys with huge guts and crap in their coronary arteries pushing their lawn mowers in the heat around their acre-and-a-half yards. Stoic eighty-year-old Scandinavians deciding it was time to climb their twenty-foot ladders and clean the old moss off their roofs.

Jason was my partner. We chatted with the off-going crew, lingering over our coffee in the sturdy firehouse kitchen. Eventually we strolled out into the fine summer sunlight, across a short expanse of pavement, and under the main rotor to check the helicopter and our medical bags for completeness and readiness. Everything looked good. No blood splatters on anything, maybe just a couple of small things missing, and we replaced them. At the time, I had been a flight nurse for about three and a half years. Jason had just transferred from another base; I'd met him and talked to him at meetings, but we hadn't flown together before. He was our youngest flight nurse, about fifteen years younger than me, which is to say he was fifteen years younger than most of us, a thing he was teased about occasionally. He was short and compact, bespectacled, analytical and smart, calm. We finished our checklists and went into the office to fax our supply requests to the main base.

Jason put his feet up on the desk and said it was almost a year to the day since he'd started with our outfit. "My first flight," he said, chuckling, "was CPR in progress for thirty minutes in the aircraft."

"Ouch! Was it trauma?"

"Yup. A rollover on the freeway. It was . . . stressful."

"Was CPR already in progress when you took over the care of the patient?"

"Yup."

"Hah! That is stressful, especially for a first flight," I said, picturing it and laughing a little. On your first-ever flight, the rush of foreign sensations—the vibration, the roar, the cramped quarters, the whizzing landscape—makes the simple act of strapping yourself in to the helicopter enough of a challenge.

"But to my mind it's not the most stressful situation," I added. "I mean, when you get trauma patients with CPR in progress, yes, it's an exercise in doing everything possible, but they're basically dead already. You can't hurt 'em."

At that point, I was thinking of a physician friend, my own gastroenterologist. I see him for gastroesophageal reflux—chronic heartburn, and who knows whether it's because of genetics, the two ten-pound babies I've borne that mashed my insides to a pulp, or this job. He told me once that when he'd first started out in medicine, he was scared to take care of really sick—critical—patients.

"But then I realized," he'd confided, grinning a little, "that they only get *so* sick, and then they die."

Yeah.

"The *most* stressful situation," I mused aloud to Jason, "is when they're lying there talking to you and *then* they code. The ones who roll back their eyes and die right there."

I can't remember if I mentioned to Jason that it was a situation that had never yet happened to me in flight, but it hadn't. And for all my years of experience on the ground and in the air, I didn't know how well I would acquit myself if it did.

I must have temporarily lost my mind, saying such a thing with that fatalism sitting like a stone in my stomach, with the twenty-four-hour day so early in gestation and our flight suits so clean, with the caffeine of the morning coffee still running in our veins. Saying such a thing on a Friday in summer.

Jason snorted. The harsh fluorescent light on the office ceiling flashed off his stylish little glasses, and I couldn't tell what he was thinking. It was probably something like *Now she's cooked our goose.* "Well, yeah," he said. "No question about it. That would be the worst."

It was early afternoon when the pager shrieked for the first flight of the day. We kicked off our sandals and zipped up our boots and our flight suits, and off we went to a small community hospital, a thirty-minute flight toward the coast, over open valleys and rivers winking like bottle caps in the hot noonday sun. Brad, our pilot, dropped the aircraft down light and easy onto the helipad, and Jason and I slid our stretcher, bags, and monitor out onto a gurney. We trucked the whole thing in through the emergency department door and up to the ICU on the second floor.

Our patient was Doug. He was forty-six years old, with esophageal cancer and an upper gastrointestinal hemorrhage, and we were transporting him to an oncology referral center, where they had more resources to deal with his problems. His esophagus, which transports food from the mouth to the stomach, had a large tumor on it, and he had been receiving chemotherapy and radiation to debulk it, to shrink it enough so that a surgeon would have a shot at removing it. Apparently, a blood vessel in that region had eroded earlier that morning. It had gouted large amounts of blood.

A hematocrit measures the percentage of the volume of red blood cells in the total volume of blood and is used as quick guide to how much blood has been lost and how well it's being replaced. A normal crit is about 40 percent. After he started vomiting blood, Doug had an initial crit of 17 percent. He had received five units of packed red blood cells and other blood products since that measurement had been taken, but there hadn't been a repeat crit. He had not vomited any blood recently, and he came with a tube that had been surgically placed in his stomach through his abdominal wall—there wasn't much output from that, either. We could assume that the bleeding vessel had clotted off. For the moment.

He had other problems too. A collection of straw-colored fluid between his left lung and the pleura, the covering around his lung: a pleural effusion caused by impaired lymphatic drainage secondary to his tumor. The ICU staff had just drained 520cc—more than two cups, quite a bit. I hoped it wouldn't reaccumulate too quickly. He also had a small pneumothorax of the right lung. This was a collection of air between the pleura and the lung. The problem for us was Boyle's law: air expands at altitude, and aloft a small pneumothorax can become a large pneumothorax, collapsing the lung and, if it's big enough, compressing the heart and the great vessels that transport blood into and out of the heart. In an ICU, a big pneumo would buy the patient a chest tube so air could drain continuously. At altitude, if it became a problem, Jason and I would temporarily treat the pneumo with a flutter valve—a large-bore, sharp steel needle that had been sterilized with a disposable-glove finger rubber-banded to the hub. The glove finger acts as a one-way valve. We'd stick the needle through his chest wall, into the space between the second and third rib, and it would allow air to escape.

And there at hell's heart, Doug just *looked* end-stage. Esophageal cancer tends to be advanced by the time it announces itself. He was skin and bones, shadowed hollows instead of mounded pink flesh, a victim of his own personal holocaust. His hair and eyes were brown, but he was so ashen an Impressionist would paint him in shades of gray.

He was, however, awake and alert, polite and pleasant, exhibiting the prosaic courage of an ordinary person in an extraordinary situation, the sort of courage that redeems the human race over and over again, a million times a day. He had three or four children visiting him, a gaggle of pretty girls in their pre-teens and early teens, their midriffs showing, acid-washed jeans low on their slim hips. As I worked fast to get my equipment on him, I heard him kiss them good-bye, heard them tell him they loved him, heard him say he'd see them later.

Jason had finished taking a report from the ICU doc out at the nurses' station desk. We were almost ready to go. I took stock of Doug's vital signs on the monitor over his bed. He had a decent blood pressure for the moment and a low-normal oxygen saturation, but his heart rate and respiratory rate were high, and it was difficult to tell exactly why. It was likely he needed more blood products. His pleural effusion might have been starting to reaccumulate, or his pneumo might have started to enlarge.

I wondered if we should place a tube in his trachea before transporting. This would allow us to breathe for him, to take control of his airway and maximize his oxygenation and ventilation. The reasons for doing it were obvious—he was skating close to the edge, on the verge of decompensating. It's easier to intubate in the ICU with five people to help than in the aircraft, and it'd be one fewer set of problems for us to deal with if we ran into trouble en route.

But intubation would take time and delay transport. And even with the muscle relaxants and sedation that are used to accomplish the procedure in a conscious patient, it can cause a spike in blood pressure, a spike that could blow a barely formed clot off an esophageal blood vessel. The question for us was whether Doug's tenuous situation would maintain itself for the hour that it would take to reach the large referral center. It was a judgment call.

"His respiratory rate is twenty-eight," I murmured to Jason. Normal is about twelve. I was on the fence about intubation, and I could see that Jason was too. I shrugged, to let him know I was equivocal. He waggled his head from side to side. We both sneaked a glance at Doug. He was still hugging his girls and chatting with the ICU nurse. Jason and I wrinkled our noses, shook our heads. Without a word passing between us, we decided we'd just get out of Dodge.

Probably thinking of the esophageal cancer at the base of this mess, an illness that was likely to be terminal, Jason turned to Doug and surprised me by asking if he had an advance directive, a living will.

Doug said no, he didn't.

The question is certainly reasonable in and of itself, but in our practice setting, if they're calling for an emergency helicopter transport, then the patient is usually not ready to die. We can assume he's not willing to go out without some fireworks. But Jason persisted. "If something happens during the flight, do you want us to put a tube in and breathe for you? Do you want us to give you drugs?"

"Yes," Doug said. He took the questions in stride. "Do everything."

The exchange was a model of clarity.

We slid him onto the gurney, wrapped him up in our bright yellow pack, trundled out to the helipad. As we were loading Doug into the cramped confines of the cabin, he complained of stomach pain. I promised him morphine once we got settled and pushed the button on our monitor to cycle a blood pressure. The digital number clicked onto the screen—80 systolic. I felt a little worm of worry creep up the back of my neck; I increased his IV fluids as we stowed everything. I told him his blood pressure was a little low, that I was giving him a fluid bolus, that his pressure needed to improve and stay improved before I could give him anything for pain but that I'd do it as soon as I could. Narcotics drop blood pressure.

Jason settled into his right-side, aft-facing seat. I strapped myself in, facing forward on the left. The next blood pressure, gotten as we were taking off, was 110 systolic. Better. I began to breathe a little easier. The emerald valley floor slid by beneath us under a white-hot sky. Doug lay on the stretcher with his head just above and in front of me, the back of the stretcher ratcheted up at a thirty-degree angle. He seemed to be looking at the scenery.

Five minutes into the flight, forty minutes out from the receiving hospital, he started spitting at my window, saliva mixed with streaks of blood. It rolled down the Plexiglas. I reached up with the Yankauer, a rigid suction device, and tried without much success to help him use it. He wasn't paying attention. *Splu-ee.* He continued to spit at my window as if I weren't there. I lifted one of the earmuffs we had placed on him to protect him from the roar of the engines and asked him if he was okay. He nodded yes. He wasn't retching, just spitting.

But then he urped up a glob of frank blood (*That was our clot,* my mind whispered) that landed on the floor next to my left boot, and before another thought could cross my mind, he was unresponsive and apparently seizing. His jaw was clenched, his eyes were closed and twitching (*rolled back his eyes*), and he started to spout blood out of his nose and mouth. It was thin, watery blood, as if the hematocrit was low. Very low.

He still had a blood pressure, 140 systolic. A heart rate in the 140s as well—high, his heart pounding away, trying to make too few blood cells do all the work. But the shit was hitting the fan, no question about it. We increased his IV fluid again, and

Jason wrapped a pressure bag around the single unit of packed red blood cells that the sending hospital had been able to give us. They had used most of their stock of red cells on Doug earlier in the day. Jason and I knew we had to intubate him, and while we were pawing at the respiratory bag and pulling out the supplies, his heart rate and oxygen saturation dropped into the sixties. This is one step away from dying outright.

"Fuck," I said, and Jason agreed.

Our pilot asked what was happening. He had been a paramedic, and he could hear our terse exchanges over the intercom.

"He's going down the tubes," I said. "This is going to *suck*. We're both out of our seat belts." We let the pilot know when we're unrestrained, so he can avoid unexpected maneuvers.

"Got it." He asked us if we wanted to divert to the trauma center. This was a good idea. The trauma center had a helipad; it was ten minutes closer. The trauma center was also a little more geared up for this sort of emergency.

Using a mask and bag to breathe for Doug, we bagged both his heart rate and oxygen saturations up to near normal levels. The nurse sitting on the left side in our aircraft is in the airway-management seat. A successful intubation is all about getting a good view of the vocal cords, and the ergonomics for intubation are a little better from the left.

That meant me. Making a mental and physical effort to keep tabs on my equipment, which wanted to scatter all over the floor, I edged over from the left seat to the middle of the cabin while Jason continued to ventilate with the bag and mask. I wedged myself between the monitor/defibrillator and the head of the stretcher. My butt rested on the monitor screen. As makeshift and uncontrolled as it sounds, this position worked pretty well for me. It was probably ninety or even a hundred degrees in the helicopter, and I'm sure I was sweating buckets, but I don't remember my body at all. I slid the laryngoscope into Doug's mouth with my left hand. The scope has a blade to keep the tongue out of the way, and a bright light at the end of the blade so you can see what you're doing. Blood kept welling up into his airway from his esophagus, and I had to suction him several times with my right hand before I got a clear view of his vocal cords. But there they were, pearly white. I had less than a second to drop the suction catheter, pick up the ET tube, and slide the tube through the cords before blood fouled the field again. But he had stopped seizing, and he was anatomically easy to intubate. I knew I was in. Even under those circumstances, there was a subintellectual pleasure in it.

Unfortunately, by this time, he had also lost any semblance of a heart rate. A flat line, asystole (*die right there*). I uttered the word *fuck* a few more times into my headset, alternating it with *shit* occasionally. Jason started chest compressions, and he did them with his elbow as he pushed some atropine and epinephrine, drugs that stimulate an unresponsive heart. I bagged Doug through the tube with 100 percent oxygen, but it didn't improve his heart rate at all. And it was hard to bag him, harder than it should have been. I could see his chest rise, but of course with the engine noise we couldn't listen for lung sounds, which is one way to confirm that the tube is in the right place. We put a carbon dioxide detector in-line, another way to confirm. It registered a low level of carbon dioxide. This meant one of two things: either we were in the wrong place, in his esophagus, picking up some gas from his stomach, or we were in the trachea but he was so far gone his lungs weren't exchanging much carbon dioxide.

In case our 1,500 feet of altitude and positive-pressure ventilation had turned Doug's small right-lung pneumothorax into a big pneumothorax, Jason stuck a flutter valve in the upper right chest. It didn't improve things.

We decided to re-intubate. I thought my original tube was good. It was pretty clear that Doug was exsanguinating, bleeding out, and that was the cause of all our woes. But if the tube happened to be in the esophagus instead of the trachea, then Doug wasn't getting any oxygen, and we were hosed. It was the same deal as before—suction several times, go for it during the one-second window while Doug's throat was clear of blood. As before, I saw the tube slip right through the vocal cords. We left this tube in. We were still at least twenty minutes away from landing, suspended in a bubble of blood and sweat over an anonymous verdant landscape. Doug's pupils had gone fixed and dilated, more evidence that he was *dead right there.*

I craned my head toward the door on the left as I bagged breaths into Doug, trying to work out the kink in my neck from the unnatural posture of intubation. It was then that I saw the tiny lightning crack of sky. It limned the worn gray vinyl that lined both door and frame: my door was ajar. It hissed high and tight with 160 knots of disturbed airflow.

I was still out of my seat belt. I had bounced around untethered in the cabin for more than ten minutes. I would have sworn the door was secure when we lifted off the helipad; I double-check it every time. I didn't remember hitting the door handle at all in flight. But bags and equipment (and our elbows and knees) had been knocking around the tiny cabin and maybe something had hit it, or I'd hit it, and in my ultra-focused, out-of-body state, I hadn't noticed. If I had been the one doing chest compressions instead of Jason, I would have wedged my ass against the door to get enough leverage. (A practice I have since abandoned. No need to become a hole in the ground in some bucolic backwater.)

I couldn't latch the door shut. The aerodynamics of flight prevented it. And as long as we're flying straight at speed, the pilots say, it can't open. This should have been a comforting fact, but my gut had trouble accepting the truth of it, so I put my seat belt back on, cinched it tight, breathed for Doug with my right hand, and gripped the door handle with my left.

When a patient goes into cardiac arrest in an ER or an ICU, a mass of highly educated people converge to help. Jason and I were alone. We had started with four hands between us to run a full resuscitation, and now we had only three. The whole situation had degenerated so outrageously it started to feel like comedy.

"Brad," I said to the pilot, "my door's open, for chrissake! I'm buckled back in. Try not to bank left, will you?"

He laughed outright, unperturbed. "Well, you're just not having a good day," he said. He sounded cheerful.

But at least we had bottomed out. We continued to give fluid through two large-bore IV lines, using up our entire supply, but we had no more blood products to give. Jason kept up chest compressions and pushed epinephrine at appropriate intervals. I bagged and held on to my door. We asked Brad to radio for paramedics to meet us at the trauma center's helipad. As soon as it was logistically possible, we wanted more than three hands to work with.

The end of the story is predictable. Experienced urban medics met us out on the blazing concrete of the pad the second we shut down. One of them checked my tube placement and deemed it good. Our flutter valve was dislodged as we all pulled Doug out of the aircraft. Since we could finally hear breath sounds and could tell they were decreased over Doug's right lung, we knew we needed to put it right back in. His breath sounds on that side improved immediately thereafter.

But his pupils remained fixed and dilated, his gray face streaked with his watery blood. The ER staff—and surgeons, gastroenterologists, nurses, respiratory therapists, anesthesiologists, social workers, unit secretaries, and our medical director—descended on us as soon as we rolled in the door. They had a blood bank full of red cells and a rapid infuser; against what I considered significant odds, they got his heart beating again for a little while. But Doug arrested again (*died*) within an hour, while he was in the CT scanner and we were standing in the ER trying to reconstruct the minutiae of the flight and put it on paper. There were speculations of an esophageal tear, but I never did hear the actual autopsy results. I don't know exactly what went wrong in the red darkness of Doug's gut.

"You and I had that conversation this morning . . . ," Jason said as we huffed our way out to the pad with our loaded, freshly remade stretcher.

"Weird," I agreed. "And you asked him if he had an advance directive . . ."

We still had eighteen hours to go and four more flights ahead of us, and when the pager went off for the last one, at seven the following morning, it took us right back out to the same small hospital where we (*Doug*) had started. A middle-aged man again, a car accident this time. A complicated pelvic fracture for sure. Possible aortic trauma. We had to balance adequate fluid resuscitation against the possibility of blowing out a weak spot in our patient's aorta. The whole night had been like that. It was a shift dogged by the specter of exsanguinations.

I couldn't think about Doug until I was on my way home, two hours late and near catatonic with exhaustion. I drove seventy-five miles through the fading cool of late morning, the blond fields of a Saturday in summer streaking away on both sides of the highway. Maybe I blasted the B-52's, or maybe I was too tired.

I thought about a third IV line we could have placed. I thought about blood products we didn't have. I thought about Doug's daughters and their poignant good-byes. I hoped they didn't think we'd killed him, as I might have in their place. After all, he was still alive, still talking—he was still their dad when Jason and I rolled him away.

And I wondered where Doug's daughters were when he died. I still picture them like this: chattering in a car somewhere between the coast and the city, on a rural road that shimmers with August heat. They wind through a dense sea of trees—cedars, hemlocks, masses of blowsy maples in full leaf but somewhat past their prime. Our aircraft crosses over them. The brief shadow we cast on their landscape is fraught with something, a startle or a blessing.

Chapter Two

A Hold on the Earth

I know I will not remember her name.

I remember instead the labels attached to her: *Ichthyosis. Hydrocephalus.* Looking back, I realize there was probably some error in her very fabric. There's a text, *Smith's Recognizable Patterns of Human Malformation,* that I think of as the syndrome bible: nearly a thousand pages on what happens when the most basic stuff of a body goes wrong. There are pictures of malformed babies and children, hundreds of them, all with black marks, like blindfolds, over their eyes. Protection of their privacy, their identities. But there is also the prurient eye of the camera, recording the places where the coding of a human being stumbles. Where cells, multiplying one by one in the darkness of a womb, branch away from the well-lit, well-provisioned road of normality.

I loved the language of medicine from the first, and I still love it—the precision of it, the way it gives shape to chaos. If I look up *ichthyosis* and *hydrocephalus* in *Recognizable Patterns,* I may find some imperfect understanding of where her cells failed her. I may find a photo of a baby with an immense head, a wasted body, and the skin of a fish, along with a bloodless description of how such a baby might come to be in the world. I would take comfort in it. The language of medicine names the unspeakable, and moves on.

Yet her name is all she had to announce herself, and I've forgotten it. That feels like failure.

I can see her, though. The fine scattering of reddish hair that covered her huge, fluid-filled head, the dilated blue of her veins mapping out her scalp. I see how the bones of her skull were like islands, separated by wide straits of soft tissue. And I see the scales that covered every inch of her, except for the palms of her hands and the soles of her feet. Scales that flicked off, left raw and bleeding places, if I rushed with the washcloth when I changed her diaper. Dead scales that sloughed off in her incubator. She was a sacrifice for a primitive god, pinned on her slab by the sheer mass of her head. Entranced and alone behind the translucent leavings of her skin, a halo made of insect wings.

And I have muscle memory of her: the medicine-ball weight of her head in the crook of my left arm, the sweet hint of her body lying across me as I rocked her. Half of each iris was sunk below the rim of each lower lid, forced down by the pressure in her head. There was no way to tell for sure what lay behind the gray half-moons of her eyes, what thought or absence of thought. She cried in infrequent, weird bursts that trailed off, like the clatter from a windup toy. I know now, from scores of babies that came after her, that it was a neurogenic cry, an emblem of brain malformation or damage. When I hear something like it now, twenty-seven years later, I know right away how much is wrong that no one can fix.

But she was able to take comfort, my little pea. Her eyelashes were red and sparse, like her hair, and she blinked faster, more ostentatiously, it seemed, when she was happy. When I held her, she settled in, turned toward my warmth with hers. Her own heat was so slight, like her hold on the earth.

By CT scan, her brain was grossly abnormal. I remember that her family stopped visiting after her first few days of life, expecting her to die, and that there were plans for institutionalization as the weeks went on. And institutions conjured the image of some Dickensian orphanage, even as late as 1979.

I remember wishing, in my unformed, twenty-one-year-old way, that I could adopt her. Someone, I thought, should be able to save a brand-new baby from becoming a forgotten cog in an institutional wheel. Wasn't that a given? I was fresh from the nursing homes I had worked in during my undergraduate days, where spirits in an unknown state of grace or damnation were frozen in hellish, twisted bodies. That setting seemed all wrong for someone with the clean slate of a newborn, someone who had so recently arrived in this life.

I remember the day I came to work and saw her incubator was empty, like a lung that had just exhaled.

But that isn't the whole story.

I know that the more experienced nurses on the unit didn't share my soft spot for her. They cared for her with economical movements, the casual grace of expertise, but they turned their inner gaze from her, females of a herd refusing to feed an orphaned runt.

"Why do you hold her all the time?" Karen asked me one evening as I sat with the baby in our accustomed place, the scarred wooden rocker in front of the Isolette. Karen was smiling, teasing me. The little pea and I traced a section of institutional flooring over and over, slow and measured, back and forth. Karen was about fifteen years older than I was, and she had spent at least ten of those years in that place, the neurology/neurosurgery unit of a large children's hospital. A few nurses there had desiccated into wasps, penetrating but venomous. Karen wasn't one of those. It was just that she was hundreds of brain-damaged babies, thousands of tragic stories ahead of me.

"You've seen that baby's CT scan. You know she has about as much brainpower as an earthworm," she said, chuckling.

I could feel the little pea's pale fire against me, right over my heart, but at the same time, rising on my inner screen like a vision, was the earthworm I had dissected in tenth grade: one nerve running up the length of its body, bifurcating at its head into a simple *Y*. The *Y* is its "brain." Nothing is much more basic than the brain of an earthworm.

I snorted back a laugh. I'm still not sure if that laugh was salvation or damnation. But I do know that when you take a scalpel to the nervous system of an earthworm, the trick, then as now, is to expose that tender bifurcation without destroying it.

∾

Decades later—after my practice environment had transitioned through multiple neonatal and pediatric intensive-care units and morphed from a scarred rocking chair to the back of a helicopter—my partner and I, along with our patient, would whirl around at the start of each flight, turning on and plugging in equipment during the two or three minutes it took for the pilot to power us up for takeoff. We would be parked on a rooftop helipad, in a field, or on the surface of a vacant lot/freeway/airport, and once the rotors were spinning so fast they were invisible, once we could feel the roar/whine/vibration build to a crescendo in our bones, we were ready to go. At that point, our pilot would radio our dispatcher and the airport tower to call us off. Along with a brief, patterned description that might include our call sign, tail number, location, and destination, he would state the number of occupants in the aircraft. One pilot had a particular way of phrasing it, a fragment of poetry in a technical paragraph of aviation-speak, and it never failed to catch my ear.

"Four souls aboard," he would say. Then he'd lift us toward the sky.

And every time he said it, I felt the random weight of the world press in on our small bubble of aluminum and Plexiglas. Every time, I pictured our craft as if I were floating alongside it, looking in through the window at our four tiny heads bent to our work—and our fates—improbably suspended in midair. I usually thought, too, of my little family of four: my husband, Howard, my sons, Kieran and Gabe. It was a matter of chance on both scores that the four of us, four souls out of billions on the planet, had come together for a brief passage through time and space. In the helicopter, there was plenty to do and no time to dither. Yet every time our pilot called us off that way, I saw with resigned clarity—and an involuntary upwelling of tenderness—how fragile we all were.

Chapter Three

Omens

A dark, rainy mid-December.

My younger son, Gabriel, was a tight knot of cells I wasn't even aware of yet, conceived the previous weekend in Los Angeles, where Howie and I had gone for his company Christmas party.

I was the oldest of a family of five, and by then had been a neonatal/pediatric ICU nurse for nearly a decade. Even before I had children of my own, perhaps especially before I had children of my own, I thought of myself as a maternal pro. Having seen the worst on the units, having had a hand from a very early age in mothering the four kids born right after me, I had a light touch with parenting. And right from the beginning, Kieran, a huge blond infant born two years earlier, had been an easy baby, good company. There was something companionable about him, a we're-in-this-together quality. He was a cheerful talker even before he could produce an intelligible sentence. But ever since Kieran had joined us, the thought of a second child had produced cold sweat and night panic. I was shocked at the intensity of it: *not ready, not ready.*

Over the previous six months, some rigid antigestation security guard had finally relaxed. The shape of a second child had begun to coalesce.

Back at work, in the pediatric intensive-care unit of a large urban medical center, my patient was a twelve-year-old boy from a Filipino family. He had begun to exhibit bizarre behavior at home and was admitted to the unit with a decreased level of consciousness. He was intubated and placed on a ventilator. With all kinds of arcane tests coming up negative, he had progressed straight through to brain death within a few days. I had taken him down for the study that showed there was no blood flow to his brain. Massive brain swelling had completely cut off circulation, and only after an autopsy did we learn that the cause was rabies, and, judging from the strain of rabies, the vector was a bat. Rabies had been overlooked because there was no known history of a bite, from a bat or any other creature. Usually an animal bite is a significant event, and parents remember it. If they know about it.

Rabies is almost uniformly fatal once symptoms develop. The U.S. Centers for Disease Control and Prevention states that during the period 1990 to 2007, thirty-four naturally acquired bat-associated human cases of rabies were reported in the United States. A bite was reported in only six cases. Seventeen cases documented physical contact with a bat in the home or workplace, two with a possible bite, fifteen with no recollection or knowledge of a bite. And in eleven cases, no bat encounter was reported at all.

If my young patient had sustained a bite, he failed to mention it to his family. Maybe he was someplace he wasn't supposed to be when he was bitten, messing around in somebody's old attic or garage or under some graffiti-defaced urban bridge where bats liked to roost. And he had gone camping a month or two prior to presenting with symptoms; he'd slept outdoors in an area where bats were known to be endemic. Bat bites, reportedly, can be painless. The theory was he'd been bitten in his sleep.

I've tried to picture this scene, and I always fail. A church group's allotment of kids, say, huddled in sleeping bags under an impassive sweep of black sky. The ultrasonic phase-shift of rubbery wings, roiling the air next to the sweet cheek of some mother's son. As needle teeth sink down into a neck or a face or an arm or a hand, wouldn't they disturb even the deepest sleep of the most untroubled childhood?

The CDC reports that there has never been a cluster of cases associated with a group of campers. One rabid bat, then— one wanton, imperceptible moment of penetration.

And I can still see the boy's saliva all over my bare hands. Six years into the HIV odyssey, and I still wasn't as glove-conscious as I should have been. My hands were flaky and excoriated from constant hand washing. How many breaks in the skin of my hands? How many microscopic open sores, just the right size for a rhabdovirus to slide through? His secretions flowed steady; radioactive lava oozing out of his mouth and nose. Gallons of saliva loaded with rabies virus, so much you couldn't keep him dry even if you suctioned him every five minutes.

On our return from the cerebral-blood-flow study, when the elevator dinged and the door trundled opened on the PICU floor, his mother was waiting for me. She was small, brown, watchful. Wings of black hair framed her face. With one hand and a knee, I manhandled the heavy bed to a stop in front of her, in the hall just outside the main doors of the unit; with the other hand I manually breathed for her son with a bag attached to an oxygen tank.

What did the test show, Jennifer?
I think you should sit down and talk with the doctors.
You know what it showed. I can see it in your eyes.

They're nothing if not straight shooters, Filipino mothers. I heard strains of Martha Reeves and the Vandellas: *Nowhere to run to, baby. Nowhere to hide.*

There's no blood flow to his brain at all.
He's dead, then, Jennifer.
Yes. I'm so sorry.

She dropped to her knees, right there in the hallway in front of the PICU entrance, and began to keen. There is no other word for it. It was a piercing, mournful, dreadful, mind-altering sound, and on the fifth floor of a busy medical center one dark December, it froze motion and stopped time.

December turned to January. Gabe and I received the rabies series, five deep intramuscular injections beginning the day we learned the autopsy results and continuing on through days 3, 7, 14, and 28. I was in my first trimester; Gabe's organs were forming. I called my obstetrician to explain the situation and to ask her if anything was known about the effects of the vaccine during organogenesis, and she said, "Well, nothing is worse than rabies!" And I had to laugh.

Throughout the soft spring that followed, I ran almost every day. I still believed in God then. The repetitive motion of exercise was—still is—meditative for me, and I sometimes prayed as I ran. But I prayed divided: half with a form of hope and surrender to a larger consciousness that surged in fits and starts, and half with a cool stillness that inhaled the astringent scent of the eucalyptus trees on my footpath, a stillness that waited and watched and didn't give any quarter to concepts like gods or virgins or miracles. That half needed evidence more than it craved hope, and I believed then what I believe now: that we are organic beings, easily disrupted or destroyed, and we are neither more nor less important than all the other organic entities of this world. We are protoplasm, which I believe is perhaps the same as saying: *we are stardust.*

———

It had been a busy day. I'd just given report to another nurse on the patient I cared for that morning, a baby with a newly repaired congenital heart defect, and I hadn't had any lunch. Gabe and I were both a little bitter about that. As I hustled down the hall toward them, Joanna was staring into the dark space above the unit secretary's head. She hopped from one foot to the other and fidgeted with her hands, much the way the little pip inside me would do throughout his life. She was four years old, a wisp of a person. All eyes, not much hair. Her scalp gleamed through the fragile black fuzz growing back after her last course of chemo.

As with any admission, I knew a few advance facts about her. Acute lymphoblastic leukemia—ALL—and she had already re-lapsed after one bone-marrow transplant. This would be her second. It wasn't quite conscious—twenty other things com-peted for my attention—but my gut twisted a little as it calcu-lated her chances of surviving her cancer and thriving.

For Joanna's second transplant, the donor marrow was to be surgically sucked from the hips of her sister, a different sis-ter this time than for her previous transplant. But first, over the upcoming days before transplant day, chemo and radiation would obliterate her own bone marrow and, along with it, her leukemia. At least, that was the plan.

Bone marrow, however, produces blood cells. Red blood cells carry oxygen. White blood cells fight infection. Platelets clot wounds. As we destroyed her own marrow and during the wait for her sister's marrow to engraft and to begin producing blood cells, infection could kill her. She would become anemic, exhausted. She'd develop bruises and the potential for hem-orrhage. In her immediate future, then, would come chemo, radiation, dozens of blood products, and potent IV drugs like antibiotics and antifungals, so many there was barely enough time in a twenty-four-hour day to infuse them all.

Sores would open up from her mouth right through to her intestines. She wouldn't eat for weeks. There'd be omnipresent nausea, bottom-scraping vomiting—scant teaspoons of stomach acid and bile. Constant diarrhea. Four times a day, we would ask her to swallow antibiotics that tasted like motor oil mixed in cherry syrup, an attempt to prevent the normal bacterial flora of her gastrointestinal tract from burgeoning into an overwhelming, life-ending infection. One bone-marrow-transplant patient from our center had died in that manner, and it altered our practice—the antibiotics were an attempt to prevent it from happening again. But Joanna, like all of our BMT patients, would retch up this concoction repeatedly. We were supposed to re-feed it, as ridiculous as *that* sounds. I don't think many of us did it.

As I walked down the hall toward her, I tried to gauge the expression on her face. *Pensive* described it. Sober. She was scared, I decided. Well, who wouldn't be? She'd been through the whole vicious process once before. She knew the score. These were her last few minutes in the outside world. I would walk her down the hall, the door of her high-cleaned laminar-flow room would click shut behind her, and there she would stay until the marrow of sister number two floated to the center of her small skeleton and made itself at home.

Ten days of radiation and chemical poison, a bag of her sister's bone marrow or an infusion of stem cells derived from it—I can no longer remember which—and then the long, breathless wait for her cell count, her absolute neutrophil count, to rise like a phoenix from the ashes. Three to four weeks in the room, probably more. And submerged beneath the surface of the days, like an undertow, the thought that she might never leave it.

There's no way to put a good spin on any of this, I was thinking. I reached out and touched her shoulder, startling her, and she looked up, her dark eyes huge.

Something in me braced itself, as for impact. I would be spending all my workdays with her for as long as it took.

"Hi, Joanna," I said. "I'm Jennifer. I'm going to be your nurse." I bent down to shake her hand. Gabe was too small yet to impede me.

But then she grinned. Her teeth—still baby teeth, after all —were a flash of surprise in the brown of her face. Her eyes crinkled up at the corners.

"Jenneefa," she said. "I'm happy to meet you." She covered my hand with both of hers. They were tiny but warm. It was a gesture she shared with her mother, Verna, who was standing next to her but excused herself to take care of some admission paperwork downstairs.

I didn't expect her easy camaraderie, her good humor, but I knew how to run with it. I wished my social skills were half as good as hers. I picked up her belongings and we ambled down the hall. Joanna leaned in, her head at my waist. She chattered about the new toys in her bag, all bright plastic that could be wiped down with antiseptic solutions. She told me all about her brothers and sisters. They were a large Catholic family, which is a good thing when you need multiple transplant donors. I gowned, masked, scrubbed, and gloved as she talked, before we entered her room. Neither of us noticed the moment when the door swished shut behind us.

She changed into the sterile pajamas I gave her, still talking about her cat, and climbed up on the bed, staking it out as her personal trampoline. She got impressive loft out of a lumpy hospital mattress. The transplant rooms were set out in a row, like the rooms in a railroad flat, with windows between them, sometimes curtained for privacy, sometimes not. As she jumped, she made faces through the window at the boy in the next room, a seven- or eight-year-old who had already received his transplant and was waiting for engraftment. He was blond, with spikes of hair sticking up every which way, and the greenish pallor of the transplant process was upon him. He had just enough energy to work the controls on a video game. But he waved at Joanna and stuck out his tongue, the beginning of a muffled, mostly silent friendship across plate glass. They would never meet face to face, or at least not in our unit. He would be engrafted and discharged several weeks before Joanna's turn would come.

I bumped about in the room, setting up IVs, stowing things. Joanna whirled around in the air to face me, her sturdy little legs working the mattress, jumping, jumping.

"My mother's praying to the Virgin, Jenneefa," she confided between bounces. "She says I need a meeracle." She wasn't the least bit upset, just matter-of-fact. A tiny straight shooter with an air of expectancy, waiting to see how I would react.

A stone in my chest lurched. Time slowed. *So many people need and deserve miracles and don't get them,* I was thinking.

But I loved Joanna a little after knowing her for two hours; that counted for something, and the truth was she needed this second transplant to engraft and keep her free of leukemia in the future, which was not statistically impossible but also wasn't very likely. The aberrant white blood cells that bloomed again and again in the dark of her bones imploded early hopes for her, middle hopes, too. The endgame was upon us.

She kept jumping, waiting for me to comment. I looked her in the eye. You can't lie to a person who has one foot out over the abyss, even if she is only four years old. The stakes are too high.

"I know you do, honey," I said. *Need a miracle,* I meant. I wanted to add that we, her health-care providers, would try our best to make the miracle happen, but none of those words would move from my gut to my mouth. The two ideas felt as immiscible as olive oil and water; the idea of a successful transplant with no relapse seemed to bear no relation to the concept of a miracle. I felt invisible winds moving upon the waters.

But it was good enough for Joanna. She nodded as she bounced, not once but several times, as if satisfied. As if I understood.

Weeks later, Joanna's mother rose from her bedside chair; she blocked the doorway as I turned to rush out of the room. Alarms I was responsible for were trilling and chirring outside; the sounds exploded in my own neural net. I made handle-the-alarms-for-me gestures to a colleague through the window and forced myself to stillness.

Joanna was a slight, white bundle in the bed between Verna and me, asleep. The spring in her legs was a memory. Transplant received, engraftment awaited. Neutrophil count, zero. No phoenix had as yet arisen from the ashes, and the ultrasonic phase-shift of fear stirred the close air of the room. The phoenix was overdue.

"I dreamed last night that the Virgin was holding Joanna in her arms, Jenneefa," Verna said. "What do you think it means?"

Her dark eyes—Joanna's eyes once removed—were on me above her mask, trained like gun barrels. She didn't blink. What I thought: *Uh-oh.*

What I felt: *Some version of eternity, hanging in the balance.*

What I said (knowing all the while how it could never be enough): "*If the Virgin is holding Joanna, Verna, it can't be a bad dream.*"

∞

Later that year, after the embryo that was Gabe had grown to ten pounds and was born by C-section, I had a first hint that my own protoplasm was disrupted.

I lived on the third floor of an urban walk-up at the time. One evening, I returned from some errands at about seven, only to remain in the car, parked in front of my building. I put my forehead down on the steering wheel and cried for a full fifteen minutes. I was too exhausted and dizzy to climb all those stairs.

I'd never felt that way before. It wasn't a normal exhaustion—that's what I know now. Not a normal postpartum exhaustion, even when you factored in nighttime feedings, though that's what I attributed it to. Not even a normal post-cesarean exhaustion. What I know now: I haven't felt tired in a "normal" way since.

I said to myself: *Suck it up, for chrissake.* It didn't help. I kept weeping into the olive-drab cushions of our 1975 Chevy Impala.

My apartment building teetered at the edge of the open ocean on a steep slope that ran from cliff top down to shore. The no-limits conjunction of sea and bluff and cypress and sky, the thrill-ride vertigo of living on the brink—that's what I loved about my neighborhood. On that long-ago evening, the dusk was orange and pink, with a dark beetled brow of fog lying offshore. I could taste the strong salt wind that over the course of years blows all the cypresses on the coastline into spooky, embattled shapes.

And there was Gabe. He was a fresh little bale, trussed in baby blankets, two or three weeks old. He blinked at me from his car seat in back, exuding unthinking trust and a kind of warm, Buddhist calm, a tiny Italian-Irish Buddhist with a sensuous lower lip and a few wisps of hair.

But those ten pounds at birth had turned into twelve pounds in the car seat. A wee infant, a whopping twelve-pound handicap. The thought of carrying him upstairs made my apartment seem like the summit of Mont Blanc.

Eventually I had to shoulder the diaper bag, like every mother. I stopped bawling. I gathered my personal resources: determination, stamina, Gabe. I opened the car door.

∽

Several months after I had moved on from the bone-marrow-transplant unit, my mother invited me to a May procession. She frequented a Filipino parish; she liked the simple fervor she found there, its warmth. It was as close as she could come on the West Coast to the flavor of the Italian parishes of her youth in Boston.

In the May procession, a statue of Mary, crowned with flowers, is carried aloft through the streets; parishioners follow behind, praying and singing. They carry candles.

A religious procession—it's not my thing at all. But my parents were singers, and I'd spent *my* youth in their choirs. I like to sing. And my mother had the knack of turning any outing into a good time. So the two of us lit our candles from the same votive at the church and trudged out in the wake of the statue.

As we rounded a corner, I saw Joanna. I wasn't expecting her. After she'd engrafted, after the day—the thrilling, hopeful day—that she emerged from the transplant room and I'd hugged her good-bye, I had lost track of her. But there she was, leaning out from the second-floor window of an apartment building. She was still in pajamas at two o'clock in the afternoon, watching the parade. And she still didn't have much hair; she looked tired, tiny, a little bloated. She wasn't smiling.

What I felt: *a shadow.*

"Joanna!" I yelled across the crowd. Never underestimate the numbers of Filipino parishioners who will turn out for a May procession. The atmosphere was *carnival;* it was Mardi Gras.

I saw her start, saw her scan the crowd. I waved my arms as a current of humanity swept me to the far shore of the street, but she never caught sight of me. Then she winked out of the window.

Chapter Four

Swimming in the Dark

The little man tried to die whenever I so much as *planned* to touch him. Every time I had business with him, I eased open the portholes of his incubator, trying to keep the noise and vibration down to a single soft *snick*. But he always beat me. He startled before I could lay a single gloved finger on him, and the startle alone was enough to tip him into a downward spiral. For all my efforts at stealth and silence, I might as well have been a baying hound. He was certainly starving and hollow boned, flushed from the safety of tall grass. I could picture him as a bird, blind in its panic, banging against the plate-glass window that overlooked San Francisco to the north. Straining toward a Golden Gate Park that was dreaming down below in darkness, toward the tower lights of the Golden Gate Bridge.

But in reality, he couldn't even cry—didn't have the maturity or energy. He was a tiny collection of skin and bones, resting on a pad of sheepskin in the cave of his Isolette. His skin was welted from even the most sparing application of tape. His bones were more collagen than calcium. Without foam rings and wedges for support, his head would conform to the topography of his mattress—the classic preemie toaster head.

There was a square of disposable diaper under him, a penned *16* on its outer plastic, pre-weighed so I could tell how much urine he deposited into it, one or two ccs at a time. There was no sweet curve to his buttocks; it was all pelvic bone and anus. The mass of equipment supporting him—ventilator, IV pumps, radiant warmer lights—outweighed him by a factor of a thousand.

It was 1991, and we spent only twelve hours together, a 7:00 p.m. to 7:00 a.m. shift I'd picked up for extra money. But it got to be like a game we played, the little sparrow and me. I would turn up the oxygen on his ventilator a bit, trying to get him prepped to be handled. I would inject a minuscule dose of morphine into his IV to make sure he had enough pain medication onboard. I'd goose the buttons on the portholes. At the subdued *pop* when they opened, always a little louder than the *snick* I was aiming for, his immature nervous system would give a jump, a single quick seizure. And just like that, he'd turn colors—plummeting through the familiar spectrum from pink to mottled to gray, finally settling on a funereal near-black. The peeping monitors would first slow, then shriek—the noise a dimly registered pain deep in my ear, my gesture to turn them off automatic and unconscious—as his heart rate dropped from 140 to 100 to 80 to 60. Going, going, gone.

My move. Working through the portholes, I'd take him off the ventilator, attach his breathing tube to a half-liter black rubber bag, an anesthesia bag. It had a valve on the end of it that let me control the amount of gas in the bag—and pressure in his lungs—as I gave him breaths. The gas was 100 percent oxygen. So high a concentration of oxygen would blind him if he was exposed to it long enough. It would burn out the blood vessels in his immature retinas, if he lived to tell that tale.

There'd be an aeon of time—seconds—during which he wouldn't respond. At all. Sweating, I'd experiment, getting a feel for his tiny lungs through the bag, trying to find the pattern of breaths that would turn him around. He tended to like both a fast rate and high pressures. High pressures cause lung damage over time, but again, "later" was a commodity we couldn't afford. Slowly, slowly, slowly, as we got into a sort of groove together, his heart rate would start to come up, his oxygen saturations would rise, and he'd shuttle back from the edge—from black to gray to mottled, and, eventually, to pink.

All that, and I still hadn't actually accomplished anything with him.

Some things have to be done. A baby can't sit in urine and feces until he gains weight. The little man couldn't turn himself. And every so often—as seldom as possible—I had to go in and clean out his breathing tube with a suction catheter. A near-death experience for sure, but a drying speck of mucus is plenty big enough to plug a tube only millimeters wide. He needed blood drawn so we could tell from his blood gases how well we were ventilating him, so we would know what to put in his IV, which was how he was getting the goods he needed to stay alive. I wanted to hug the pediatrics resident who threaded the arterial line into his whisper of a wrist. Without it, I'd have had to stab a vein or poke his heel with a lancet. With it, I got to siphon a little blood painlessly from a stopcock.

He needed his mother's uterus. I don't remember anymore why that particular womb had spit out this particular baby so early. It could have been a lot of things—from an intrauterine infection to a previous preterm birth to maternal cocaine use—or it could have been nothing identifiable. I didn't meet my patient's family that night, but I don't recall any family goblins raised when I got his story from the off-going nurse. I took care of more than one pregnant woman in the late eighties who'd smoked crack in the parking lot of the hospital hoping it would start labor. His mom wasn't one of those. And in any case, those women tended to have their own problems, not all of which were of their own making. Even they aren't the monsters they're made out to be. My patient's mom was probably just another hardworking woman who went into early labor for an unknowable reason.

I'd give a lot to be able to look out at the world through somebody else's eyes. I imagine that a moment or two would be enough—I don't want to be someone else; I just want the information. A few seconds of total immersion, a space of time long enough to soak up the input from someone else's nerve endings, catch the fireworks in someone else's brain. I don't know if it would be exhilarating or horrifying, but I think, for a few crystalline moments, it would make a lot of gray areas clear. And I wanted that from my little man, because I didn't feel I could reach him. He couldn't tell me anything more subtle than "I'm dying here, can you help me out?" and "Don't bother me unless you want your hand to cramp from hand-ventilating me for the next forty-five minutes." He was far too frail to be held; I couldn't access whatever skin contact could have taught me. He could talk to me only with the coarse voices of monitor alarms.

I couldn't find the *him* in him. That was disturbing. There's a stamp, or maybe it is sometimes as inchoate as a spark, that makes for that bit of difference between one human and another. Usually I look for a baby's spark through the mass of tubing, amid the peepings and hissings of the nursery. That we are each unique—that intrigues me. And it's easy to spot it when there's been world enough and time for the red hair to grow, for the chin to jut out six times a day in a characteristic stubborn way. You have to work a little harder to see it in the heat and light of the nursery, in gelatinous beings—lumps of wet clay, really—who are germinating in Isolettes or on open tables. Beings whose eyelids are still fused shut, who weigh in at about a pound each.

Or less. His birth weight, at twenty-five weeks' gestation, was 450 grams, almost one pound exactly. But he was a few weeks old already, and with his problems—immature lungs, infection, bowels that couldn't handle feeding (and those were only some of them)—he'd lost weight. That night, when I lifted all his lines off his mattress pad and pushed the button for the bed scale underneath him, he came in at 320 grams, just over eleven ounces. I've spent at least ten years of my life in intensive-care nurseries, and he is my personal blue-ribbon winner: the smallest human I've ever cared for.

It made the hairs stand up on the back of my neck. He was that negligible. That marginal.

Opinion is divided about when life begins and what it means; and opinion, among people who have seen them, also tends to be divided over whether very low birth-weight preemies are cute or not. And the two debates—one philosophical and one silly, at least on its face—are related. Those in on the "cute" debate are really asking: sweet infant or late miscarriage? I've noticed that optimists, and people who believe a life is whole at the moment of conception, are likely to look at a twenty-five-weeker and notice the perfect humanity of the hands and feet, so tiny and expressive they break your heart. Those who look at a preemie and see a sweet infant are thinking of the warm, seven-pound bundle the twenty-five-weeker could be. No cost is too high to get him there.

Pessimists, and those who think nature should sometimes be allowed to take its course, experience a preemie more as a gelid aberration than a sweet bundle. They see how huge the head is compared to the slightness of the body, see the deep purple strips that tape has torn in skin. They notice how high the settings are on the ventilator and how often the alarms are going off. They think about brain damage. They think about the tremendous cost of a single day in an intensive-care nursery, and about how many clinic visits for disadvantaged toddlers that day would buy.

∞

I grew up Irish-Italian Catholic. On a September morning in 1964, I held my parents' hands as we crossed the frost-heaved blacktop of the schoolyard at Our Lady of Assumption School in Chelsea, Massachusetts, a narrow patch dwarfed by the brooding shadow of the church, and they handed me over to Sister Therese Joseph. And on another brisk autumn morning a few weeks later, after I ate some Froot Loops for breakfast but before I walked the half-mile to the bus stop for school, my mother would tell me we were expecting another baby sister or brother.

Sister Therese was both tall and young, and her habit was Old Church, the head-to-toe, black-and-white version Ingrid Bergman wore in *The Bells of St. Mary's*. Sister Therese even had a tantalizing hint of hair, Bergman blond, peeking out from under her wimple. It was pulled so tight off her forehead I could feel her scalp ache.

But she was kind and apparently aware of how imposing a tall figure in an improbable costume can seem to a six-year-old. She took a knee next to me and my parents, yards of that mysterious, diaphanous black material swelling about her on the rough surface of the schoolyard. The huge rosary at her waist clicked and swayed in random patterns, the cross bouncing every which way as she glided down.

For my part, I gritted my teeth and braced myself. I was a small girl with an expressive face, shy with people until I got some idea of the emotional landscape, and adults were always trying to offer me a brand of patronizing comfort I didn't want. Beneath my social confusion, I wasn't afraid at all, had been dying to go to school for years. And I could read rather well. I held on to this knowledge like it was cash in my pocket. I knew it gave me a big leg up on first grade.

There was a moment in which some wordless shape of this information telegraphed between Sister Therese and me, a moment in which my parents, hovering protectively over us, didn't exist. I saw the corner of her mouth go up, a little half smile I liked the look of. She didn't hug me or pat my head. Instead, she shook my hand.

"So you're Jennifer," she said, in the manner of new colleagues meeting for the first time. "I'm glad you're going to be in my class."

It came to pass that at the opposite end of the arc of first grade, on June 1, 1965, to be exact, I was jumping rope at lunchtime with a couple of friends but without my usual enthusiasm for double Dutch. It was a blinding day, for one thing, far too hot for a woolly Catholic-school jumper and kneesocks.

I got snagged almost immediately when it was my turn to jump, and I had to go back to swinging the rope in the heat for Nancy and Katie. They jumped like automatons for what seemed like hours. This unlucky break roiled a formless sense of upset, a kind of emotional nausea, that had been brewing in my midsection all morning. I finally threw my end of the rope down, told my friends, "I quit." They watched me go with their mouths open.

Sister Therese, doing recess-monitor duty, caught this little vignette. Hunkered down by the chain-link fence, trying to pretend I didn't notice her, I watched from the corner of my eye as she made her way over to me. Her sensible black nun shoes practically stuck to the blacktop, which had softened like butter in the noon sun. I expected her to berate me for unsportsmanlike conduct. My grades for conduct were never quite as good as my grades in reading and math.

Instead, she knelt down next to me in the schoolyard once again. She was hot too, her face shiny below the white crown of the wimple. I caught a whiff of sweat, lusty and basic, emanating from the yards of black.

"That wasn't like you," she said, gesturing toward the rope. "Is something wrong?"

I was thinking that no, nothing was wrong, and was getting

ready to say so when my mouth moved of its own accord. It blurted out, "My mother is in the hospital, having a new baby." The knot in my stomach swelled, a sac of pus that would poison me if it burst. I burst into tears instead.

"Ohh," she said. Her tone was a little bit knowing, but she didn't overdo it. I was grateful for her circumspection, as cool as her wisp of blond hair—her knowledge that I valued independence over pity. She got to her feet and hugged me, though, and I was grateful for that too. I held on to her hips for a long moment, my cheek against the billows of her skirt. The material had a fine nap to it, no sheen. It was a thin, rough cotton in multiple layers.

"But having a new baby isn't sad," I said, pulling away, needing to get control of myself. "I shouldn't be sad about that."

What I didn't know how to say was this: *It's our fifth baby in seven years, if you include me. I'm just a little weary of being the oldest and most responsible, a little tired of getting used to new babies all the time. Tired of that much chaos. I'll catch a second wind about it, I think. But right this minute I don't feel up to it.*

"No," she said. "It's not sad. But it is a big change. And maybe you're a little worried about your mother."

Actually, I had never considered that giving birth might pose a danger to my mother. She went off with a big stomach practically every year, after all, and came back in a few days with a new sister, looking a bit deflated but not much worse for wear.

Still, I found myself nodding slowly. Worrying about my mother: it was a way to save face with Sister Therese, a way back to normalcy in this situation that had veered way off the course I'd intended.

"Do you want me to call your family?" Sister Therese was saying. "Maybe you'd like to go home. You're not going to miss anything here this afternoon." It was exactly what I wanted. I more than wanted it; for a shining second, I felt relief course through me. I wasn't up to addition and subtraction, the delights planned for the afternoon. I didn't feel like smiling and acquiescing, adhering to everything the social contract required. From the schoolyard, I could smell the brine lifting off the confluence of Boston Harbor and the Chelsea River, a mile or two away, working on me like an elixir. What I wanted more than anything was to cross Revere Beach, my feet burning like a firewalker's on the dry, gray sand, to wade through the muck of brown seaweed at water's edge, to fold myself inch by inch into the Atlantic. Its vastness lay fallow right across the street from the little beehive of our house. I needed to immerse myself in its cold, green quiet.

But then I realized my father was at Whidden Memorial Hospital in Everett. His mother, my nana, was in charge at our house, staying with us until our mother came home from the hospital. Nana was dealing with three toddlers, two of whom were in diapers—the old-fashioned, quilted-cloth kind with pins and rubber pants. You had to swish those diapers around in the toilet to get rid of the shit before you could wash them. That was one of my jobs, as the oldest. I had it down to a science. Our family didn't have the luxury of a diaper service.

Like most of the women in my family, Nana didn't drive. I took two city buses to get to school, a trip that took me an hour and a half each way. I could just imagine the look on Nana's no-nonsense Irish face when she got a call from my teacher asking her to pick me up because I was "a little worried about my mother." I pictured Nana trying to manhandle Bernadette, Christine, and Camille half a mile over to Northshore Road to catch the Winthrop bus, changing out at Revere Street to the Wood Island Park bus, pounding the searing pavement of

Chelsea until she and her entourage got to my school. All told, an odyssey of about a million toddler-miles, just to coddle me home.

"No, thank you, Sister," I said, wiping tears and sweat from my face. "I'm okay, really."

I'm not sure how I did get home that day. I think my Italian grandfather might have picked me up after school in his taxicab, so perhaps Sister Therese called home after all.

Maybe Grandpa just came. Once in a while, and often enough it was after I'd had a bad day, he would show up unbidden in his cab after school to save me the two buses home. I'd come out at 2:30 p.m. to find him parked across the street in front of the Toro dealer, leaning against the driver's door, his arms crossed. His love was like that: erratic, practical, and intuitive. A little spooky.

I do know for sure that when I got home, I found poor Nana in the wreck of the kitchen, dirty bowls and dishes piled high all around her, splatters of heavy cream on every surface. The mess was spectacular. She was making her own birthday cake, a strawberry shortcake, and she had just accidentally joggled the electric hand mixer while it whined away at top speed. Half-whipped cream beaded her shaggy white eyebrows, spattered her thick arms.

She was in a foul mood. Who could blame her? I tried to commiserate about the cream, but she wasn't having it, and after we'd eyed each other over the counter for a minute or two, like warriors, I steered clear of her. I could hear the ocean's impersonal *swish-swish* through the open windows, feel its breeze. It was as inaccessible at that moment as the moon.

I was gauging the mountain of crockery from across the room, wondering just how soon I'd be called to the dish drainer to dry it all, when my father telephoned, all happy with the news. A new baby, born on Nana's sixty-fifth birthday. A brother this time, Kevin Patrick. Nine pounds, one ounce.

∞

There's a poster that at one time or another has hung in a lot of intensive-care nurseries. It's a photograph of an open hand—a man's hand, from the size and bluntness of it—and a baby; a baby small enough to curl up asleep, safe inside the perimeter of fingers and palm. The baby is perfect, and in perfect repose: she has hair, and eyelashes, she has delicate curves that whisper of plenitude—of fat stores, and muscle. There are no IV lines, no ventilators. There is nothing of the ordered tumult of the nursery. The baby and her invisible protector emanate a palpable air of peace.

I cared for that baby, or one like her, when I was still a nursing student, when the neonatal intensive-care unit was a brand-new concept. She had been so stressed for so long in utero by her mother's severe toxemia (a condition that is now called pregnancy-induced hypertension) that her lungs had matured many weeks early. Toxemia had also stunted her growth—she was smaller than the norm for her gestational age. And so she came into the world at twenty-seven weeks' gestation, as small as a twenty-five-weeker but able to breathe on her own, needing only to grow enough to breast-feed and to keep herself warm.

She was perfect, too: mythic in her miniature self-containment. She cut a figure that was at once so small and so outsize, I couldn't help getting interested in neonatology. Less than two pounds, dressed in doll clothes (because it would be several years before clothes for preemies would be commercially available), and tough as nails, tried by fire before birth. Tough enough to achieve peace and repose, dreaming away in her incubator without a single artificial umbilical cord to the world outside it.

The little man, though, had slipped into this life unseasoned. He hadn't had her advantages. I left him alone as much as I could, incubating, between long bouts with the anesthesia bag, inside his warm bubble, lines and cords snaking away from every inch of his body. His fused lids had freed themselves without intervention a week or two after he was born, as they do. His eyes had opened in their own sweet time, a tiny miracle of development. Even disrupted development has its graces.

His eyeballs too moved back and forth in REM sleep. What were his dreams? He and his life were all potential—all question, no answer. He should have been swimming in the dark, fifteen weeks away from making any kind of splash in the world. Were his dreams laying down the fabric for his life? Was he building himself the framework for a bigger, stronger body? A body, for starters, that could digest milk, breathe for itself, tolerate a sudden noise, a draft of cooler air.

I ask because I sometimes think my own dreams are the precursors of my life. They're moving ahead of me in time and in some alternative space, laying down the road I'm about to travel. I dreamed of myself in a wedding dress, marrying my husband, just a few months after I met him. It wasn't a dream that pleased me; I was seventeen at the time, and he was a brash, overconfident thing, already pushing my buttons. I was too young to appreciate that a little friction can generate heat and light, or that snippets of black humor, well applied, can keep you off antidepressants. But we did marry, ten years later, after other loves—and a continent—had risen and fallen between us. After the Atlantic gave way to the Pacific.

And a dream showed me that I was pregnant with my firstborn. At the time, a month after our wedding, this information wasn't entirely welcome. But about the time I missed my period, I dreamed I saw my own uterus—open, like an anatomical drawing in longitudinal section. And lo and behold, there was a tiny fetus in it, complete with placenta and umbilical cord. Kieran.

That sense of déjà vu—it dogs me. Otherworldly scraps from the pit of the night are superimposed on the rough surface of day, and sometimes the details dovetail. I wonder about the nature of dreams. Most never come to pass—couldn't. But they all float untethered, free from the daily straitjacket of time and place, and some of them set a tone. You catch up to those in your own future as you move out over landscapes, inner and outer, near and far.

Of my little man's dreams, of course, I know nothing. I don't know if they were of darkness, or of light. We got through a night in 1991, the sparrow and me, came through to morning with 100 percent oxygen under our wings. That's what I know, and all I can say.

Chapter Five

Some Inner Planet

My redheaded friend was late. No doubt about it.

It was that time of the month. Hell, it was at least seven days *past* that time of the month.

I was shitting bricks.

It was mid-March in Girdwood, Alaska, and a dank, cutting afternoon wind was blowing snow devils under the firs in the meadow behind our cabin. The meadow massed with wildflowers in the brief, heartbreaking Alaskan summer. That was still at least three months away. But in every season, moose wandered through on a daily basis. Once in a while, there was also a black bear who shambled by without so much as a glance in my direction. Beyond the meadow, an embankment dropped down to the streambed. Crow Creek was just a few rivulets at that point, braided through gravel bars, choked under ice. A hundred yards upstream, I happened to know, a family of beavers had built an impressive dam.

I had an unobstructed view of this small piece of the Last Frontier—the old wooden outhouse didn't have a functional door. Sitting on the sparkling Styrofoam my brand-new husband had cut to fit over the dung hole, I shivered in my parka and considered, with Zen concentration, the crotch of my underpants. The faint ghosts of menses past clung to the white cotton lining, testament to the fact that my period tended to come early, when I wasn't quite expecting it. A cycle of twenty-three to twenty-seven days, instead of twenty-eight. My last splooge had started thirty-five days ago, on February 7. Ten days after our wedding.

Not so much as a smear of anything fresh, no matter how hard I squeezed my eyes shut and tried to conjure it. I mentally probed the corners of my pelvic region, hoping for cramps. Not a twinge.

A week ago, just after our arrival together in Alaska, there had been some brownish spotting, enough to make me break out a tampon, a little dizzy with relief. But nothing followed. No clots, not even a trickle.

Spotting—probably a blastocyst implanting itself in the wall of the uterus, a clinical voice in my head observed. It sounded smug as it went on to calculate an expected date of confinement: *Last menstrual period, February 7. Count back three months—November 7. Add one week and one year. You're due next November 14.*

I was a long way from white satin, string quartets, and the promises we'd exchanged in the mild winter light of northern California. But there was no time to linger, not with my ass freezing on Howard's brave new Styrofoam. I unwrapped another tampon. I knew it was wishful thinking.

The cabin was my contribution to the marriage, a dowry of sorts. It was a tumbledown, one-room affair that had its own share of Alaskan wildlife. There were squirrels nesting somewhere under the roof, and a mouse—I deluded myself with the notion that there was only one—who came out and cocked her head when I played Puccini's operas on the stereo. She especially liked "O mio babbino caro." Woodpeckers woke us when they drummed the framing members on the outside wall, just over the head of our bed. On summer evenings, it became our habit to hunt down the day's cadre of huge, slow mosquitoes that buzzed in every time we opened our door. We used our bedtime reading to whack ten or twenty of them. If we missed one and killed it in the morning instead, it left a bright smear on the whitewashed wall. Whether the blood was Howard's or mine was impossible to tell.

The cabin had electricity, so we were spared the constant work of feeding a wood stove throughout a winter that lasted eight months. It also allowed us to bask in vicarious sunshine and skimpy swimsuits via grainy late-night reruns of *Miami Vice*. But what with mice and squirrels' nests, insulation was nil, and our expensive heat radiated away to the stars. I suspect the resident rodents were also hard on the wiring, since the cabin burned down some years after we left.

There wasn't any plumbing. We lugged our water in five-gallon jugs from the tap at the local fire station, washed our dishes with water boiled on the stove, and took coin-op showers at the Laundromat. It was a great step forward when we purchased the Pak-A-Potti IV from Sears in Anchorage and I graduated from squatting over the Chock Full o'Nuts coffee can in the middle of the night, though Howard and I still wonder what possible improvements the model IV sported over models I, II, and III.

Howard and I had been married for forty-three days, but we'd known each other nearly ten years. Our relationship, until our recent nuptials, had been a tempestuous, multistate, bicoastal affair. It had always teetered between irritation and friendship, between friendship and lust, between lust and something deeper, more disturbing: a sense of responsibility to each other, and trust. It swung between the anything-goes, post-Pill, pre-AIDS college campus of the seventies and the heavy hand— the *mano della morte*, as my Italian mother used to say—of the Catholic Church of our childhoods, with all its eely strictures on a person's sex life.

Howard was loud and brash, quick-witted and far too bossy. But he also had blue-green eyes that threw off sparks, like an M-80 about to launch, and a wide, generous body, thick with the sort of muscle that lays transcontinental railroads or moves sixteen tons of coal. Muscle the artistic nerds in my family never even dreamed of. He first told me he wanted to marry me as we slow-danced at a party, a party at which I'm sure both of us drank more than our share of Genesee Cream Ale. We were both only seventeen. I laughed at him, but my hips, and my cells, took note of the heat between us, stored the knowledge somewhere deep.

Around the same time, my career was beginning. One of my first clinical experiences as a student was in a well-baby nursery, where normal newborns go after birth when their poor mothers, who have sutures from episiotomies on their bottoms and probably haven't slept well in months, need uninterrupted naps. I liked the nursery right away. All those brand-new lives, tiny people whose heads smelled sweet and who either cuddled when I picked them up, even though we were strangers to each other, or screamed with complete abandon. The caregiver-patient relationship is very direct in the nursery, no fussing with social niceties.

I didn't think of my relationship with Howard as anything serious. But when I cared for babies in the nursery and imagined a baby of my own, it was Howard I saw as a father. The image, like that early dream I had had of marrying him, was unsettling, to say the least; I always shooed it away. But still, the thing between us, whatever it was, that had begun on our third day of college in Troy, New York, followed us back and forth to our respective hometowns of Boston and New York City. It went underground for our junior and senior years, during which I took up with Howard's roommate, ostensibly breaking Howard's heart; he managed, with admirable resilience, to console himself with another woman. We didn't speak for two years.

The friendship component revived itself through letters in the fall of 1979, after we'd graduated and as I was dealing with more than one little pea with hydrocephalus. I can think of four from that year alone. One toddler had been living in a Dickensian orphanage and had never been shunted—a ventriculoperitoneal shunt, the most common type for hydrocephalus, is a surgically placed tube that drains excess fluid from the ventricles in the brain, where the fluid causes damage from increased pressure, to the empty space around the abdominal organs. Without a shunt, this toddler's head had grown unchecked since birth. By the time I met her, it was the shape and weight of a large pumpkin; to get her out of bed, you had to place her head crown-down on the floor with her neck rising out of it like a stalk. Yet she was amazing and resilient in her way. Since she couldn't lift or move her head, she'd dance around it, her body contorted to accommodate it—feet tapping on the floor, shod in the little Mary Janes and lace-trimmed anklets we bought her. She would pull up her eyelid with her finger to take a good hard look at you, an assessing look. In her literally topsy-turvy world, where nothing could ever be ergonomic, you would forever be upside down and a bit suspicious.

And there was an endless series of children with other neurologic disorders: A complete array of brain and spinal-cord tumors. Intractable seizures of unknown etiology—a preschooler who was completely normal until he was five but started seizing one day and never stopped, no matter what combination of drugs we tried. Nothing we did explained it or treated it. There was a baby with anencephaly. Most die at birth, but this one did not. I still remember the wording of the CT report: "a small amount of poorly organized brain." She was a normal infant from foot to eyebrow. Above her brows, she had an inch-wide crown of bone. The rest of her head was a large, fluid-filled, skin-covered sac that flopped down over her face if you failed to support it. Still, even with no brain to speak of, she nippled formula from a bottle; she cried whenever the sac flopped. It seemed to hurt. She lived for several months.

As it happened with so many of the children I cared for that year, she died when I wasn't at work, and when I came back and found her gone, I didn't know whether to be sad or relieved. Neither reaction seemed right. Toward the end, I could tell she was decompensating. The small curd of brain she possessed was enough to support only a few reflexes; as the months passed, and with time's inexorable, encoded press toward development, she came up short. She cried more and more often, and it sounded disorganized—more and more neurogenic, random out-of-sequence jangles from a damaged jack-in-the-box. That year, I learned how often it happens that all you can do is stand by, hold tight to small bodies or hands, and try not to judge what it all means.

I didn't share much of this with Howard in my letters. It was my writer-self who poured out onto those pages, in a medium black Flair on reams of yellow legal sheets. A form of juvenilia, you could say; an ongoing story in which I invented myself as an adult, as an intriguing, independent brunette Howard couldn't resist, and he was generous enough to play along. But something of my inner core leaked out into those letters too. And Howard, no slouch with a turn of a phrase, sent letters filled with a kind of patient, steady regard, letters I grew to rely on in that jittery time.

Lust entered into our bargain after I moved to San Francisco, where I worked three twelve-hour shifts a week in an intensive-care nursery, and Howard flew out to stay with me every few months at my little apartment at the top of Russian

Hill, on the Hyde and Beach cable-car line. It was the best of all worlds, as far as I was concerned, a neat little clockwork of hormones, fine dining, drives along the stunning California coastline. Long walks—hand in hand, hip to hip—through the neighborhoods of one of the most beautiful cities in the world. Excitement built when we were apart, peaked when we were together, and right about the time that frictions might start to emerge, it was time for him to fly home.

We flirted, as we had always done, with the idea of commitment, but in spite of the pressures of God and my own family's values, I really didn't want any part of that, though Howard insisted he did. I didn't want my life to settle, like the dregs of a keg. Howard hadn't lost any of his brashness or bossiness; I had no intention of succumbing to pressure to live a life I wasn't ready for with a man I wasn't sure about. It was not a period when I imagined children of my own.

In 1983, Howard left New York for Hagerstown, Maryland, to manage a moving-and-storage company. I took a temporary job as a traveling nurse in an ICN in Anchorage, Alaska. We had reached a stalemate with regard to our relationship. We shared a drink in the funky little bar next door to City Lights bookstore and agreed to remain friends.

My traveling assignment was supposed to last only eight weeks, but from the very first I fell in love with the immensity of Alaska. I kept extending my contract. After a few months, ripe to enter my pioneer-woman phase, wanting less of tacky Anchorage strip malls and more of the million square miles of nature around them, I moved to Girdwood.

It was, at that time, a rudimentary ski town at the foot of Mount Alyeska, and it had an apocalyptic feel, the feel of a place from *The Outer Limits*. To get there, you headed more or less southeast from Anchorage on the Seward Highway. The Seward was a tiny, beleaguered tongue of human infrastructure;

it flicked out between the churning riptides of the Turnagain Arm on the right and the glaciered peaks of the Chugach range that shot up with dizzying verticality on the left. After thirty-five miles of wilderness broken only by the minuscule hamlet of Bird and by four separate microclimates, you came to a seemingly ancient Texaco station, where you hung a left onto the Alyeska Highway and into Girdwood's narrow valley. My cabin was a few miles in, at mile 0.3 of Crow Creek Road. Crow Creek Road climbed a dusty five miles toward Crow Pass in summer; in winter, only dogs, snowmobiles, and cross-country skiers traversed beyond the first half a mile. My rent was dirt cheap, as befitted a place whose outhouse didn't even have a door.

More letters ensued between Girdwood and Hagerstown. I wrote Howard, at length and for the hundredth time, that he wasn't the guy for me. He said it didn't square with his own feelings, but he understood. This was a new note of resignation for him, a tone that had something of good-bye in it. With 4,500 miles between us, and so much water under the bridge, Howard was ready to be shut of me. If I had disappeared into the Great White North to avoid him, I might finally have achieved my goal.

But late one warm, stormy night in March, a year before I found myself staring at my underwear's stained crotch, I roiled the covers, unable to sleep. My stomach was stuffed with beef and merlot from the Double Musky, an excellent upscale Cajun restaurant that was right across the rutted dirt road from my cabin. This would have been an anomaly in the Lower 48, a fine restaurant stuck among primitive, unplumbed dwellings, but this was Alaska, and there were hungry, well-heeled skiers afoot. Pioneer Woman, she who had to schlep and boil water to wash dinner dishes, was a regular at the Musky.

What's the midnight wilderness for, if not to balm the troubled mind and the overfull stomach? I dressed in the dark and set out under the brooding lip of the ridge that overhung the northwest side of town. And by the time I'd scrambled an exhilarating two miles through sheets of rain and mounds of sodden snowdrifts, by the time I'd crossed the Seward Highway to stare at the black, silty waters of the Turnagain Arm, I'd realized it wasn't pepper steak that had been keeping me awake.

I was completely alone at the edge of the civilized universe. A creature at large in the nighttime wonder of this world, alone with mountains and the howl of storm and sea. It was a state of being I'd been aiming for without knowing it for a long time, and if I had been a different sort of woman, a she-wolf sort of woman, *I'd* have howled with the pure delight of it. But it was also true that thoughts of Howard had dogged every step of mine through the sleet. He was a part, somehow, of that moment's grand conjunction of woman, earth, and cosmos. After nine years and five states, I realized that his star had finally risen. Some inner planet had just shifted on its axis, given me its pagan blessing.

Two months, several letters, and a large number of expensive transcontinental phone calls later, I emerged from the frozen north to stay with him in Maryland. He asked me to marry him, and I accepted. I took a traveling-nurse job in Washington, D.C., as we considered our options; I kept paying rent on the Girdwood cabin. We had an incongruously elegant little wedding in San Francisco on January 28 and, forsaking all others, struck out for Alaska together on the first of March in Howard's '75 Chevy Impala.

But before we left, we spent a night at my sister Camille's apartment in Berkeley, California, three weeks or so after the wedding. She lived on the fourth floor of a building on Telegraph Avenue, near the UC Berkeley campus, high enough above the traffic and the panhandlers for the eucalyptus green of the East Bay hills to fill the windows. From a dead sleep on her living room futon, we came awake in the dark to the sound of curtains snapping in an aberrant wind, a wind that was unseasonably warm, almost tropical—a wind that roared, prowling the room like a presence. It smelled of sagebrush.

Howard reached for my hand. The arid wind was at work on our faces and we both knew, with the queer, otherworldly certainty that comes in the dead of night, that if we made love, if we opened that door, there was a life on that wind.

We still had wedding cake in my sister's freezer. We were broke and jobless, completely in flux, and I hadn't fully escaped the tentacles of the Church, by which I mean we were using the rhythm method of birth control. I was twelve days out from the last turn of the crimson tide. In the schema of the rhythm method, twelve days into a twenty-five-day cycle rates a black-and-yellow sign: Dangerous Intersection. Of *course* the egg was flaunting itself in inner space, ripe to be taken by some intrepid Culkin spermatozoon.

We looked at each other for a split second that seemed to go on forever. But then, we shrugged.

Chapter Six

A Little Taste for the Edge

The year he turned fourteen, the year before he discovered the camaraderie and muscle-bound rigor of high school football, Gabe and I often went out for fast bike rides on the local hills. These are rolling secondary roads in an area that can't decide if it's rural or suburban, routes glinting with splintered glass at the verge but overarched with hemlock and fir. The graceful arms of western cedar dip down through the brine off the inlets, providing benediction. In the homestretch of our normal loop, there's a steepish descent, half a mile long. We come to this piece of rough, chip-sealed real estate after we've humped our way up seven hills, at the point in the ride when we can smell the barn.

Both Gabe and I like speed. I take that hill with everything I'm worth, dialed into the biggest gears, pedaling for every drop of thrust I can squeeze out of bike and downgrade. I watch the driveways for cars entering the road, dimly aware I'm giving short shrift to that task. I'm down in the drops with my hands on the levers, but there's a part of me, surprisingly intractable, that would rather die than brake. For a space of seconds that seems to encapsulate eternity, I'm as free and direct as a bullet on its trajectory. There's a buzz in brain and bone at the top of the hill—perhaps it's fear, but I won't swear to it—that alchemizes into something else entirely by the bottom, something that blows unsettled dust out of every mental corner. It's a feeling suspiciously close to ecstasy.

But there's something in Gabe, a kind of fidgety restlessness, that needs to push the limits of any envelope. As a thirteen-month-old, he'd taught himself to climb out of his crib, as I discovered when he entered my bedroom and pried open my eyelid with his tiny finger. As a toddler, he'd moved kitchen chairs and climbed a pitch of countertop and shelving to reach and breach a bright bottle of something medicinal, something that nearly required the involvement of the poison control center in our lives. The bottle was twinkling, cherry red, and just under a ten-foot ceiling. Irresistible! So it isn't surprising that the year he turned fourteen, on that stretch of road, he upped the ante on our speed run. He added a little slalom to it, weaving on and off the graveled shoulder at thirty-five miles per hour, using his legs to steer a bike gone rickety from countless other stunts. His back was straight as a Viking's, his hands grasped the seat stays right below his butt. In half a mile of screaming downhill, he didn't touch the handlebars once.

Descending behind him, the pediatric ICU/emergency-transport nurse thought about a teenager's propensity for risky behavior. She thought about *mechanism*, trauma shorthand for the immutable forces and immovable objects that act on a human body at the moment of injury. Gabe's mother needed to exert authority, to scream at him to *Watch out!*, ached with the vision of a tangled mass of metal, curls, and bone gone silent in the ditch. But the hellraiser in me, of which there is a great whacking streak, never loved Gabe more than it did in those moments. Off the bike, he was gawky—a boy with huge feet like a puppy's, grown about two-thirds of the way toward a man's body. On the bike, his movements were offhand, relaxed, almost dreamy. Sure of themselves. He was a casual creature of light, an angel of proprioception at the holy coordinates where speed meets balance.

It's the stuff of cliché, but amazing nevertheless, how fast a newborn can graft into your life, how soon you can fall in love with him. If you're his biological mother, you live with him for forty weeks before he's born; he springs straight from your cells. But that's a knowledge of the viscera, not a relationship. You might or might not love the idea of him before he's born, but either way you don't really know him. That's the mystery of uniqueness, the fingerprint of the human being. Your child isn't you. Isn't his father, or his brother. But by the time I took Gabe home from the hospital, I did know he was just what our family needed. At three, our older son, Kieran, was almost relentlessly verbal. He was already a good storyteller, a master of ceremonies prone to continuous, amusing, exhausting commentary. "Millions of dollars' worth of Fords!" he would announce from his car seat as we passed a dealership. Yet for all his social skills, Kieran didn't especially like to be touched. If I held him, he wanted to sit in my lap like a sentinel on alert, facing outward to where things were happening. He cried if I tried anything too cuddly on him. Today, as a twenty-year-old, if I move to kiss him, Kieran bows his head so my kiss will land somewhere in the blond Brillo above his forehead. For him, a kiss on the cheek is too close for comfort.

Gabe was different, a relief from Kieran's merry carnival. He was quiet, ruminative—the sort of boy who looked out the window a lot, kept his thoughts to himself so much that I found myself wondering what they were. And when I held him, he nestled. He wasn't needy, didn't cry for it. He just knew how to settle into me, his lush lower lip relaxed, the first lustrous wisps of a head full of curls tucked up under my chin.

When Gabe was a few months old, I dreamed he had cancer, a particular form of cancer called rhabdomyosarcoma. In waking life, it's a solid tumor, a soft-tissue neoplasm with a number of pathologic subtypes. It can occur anywhere in the body, and the survival rate from it varies, depending on subtype and location. *Rhabdo-* is from the Greek *rhabdos*, meaning "rod." The tumor cells are rod-shaped, made up of striated muscle fibers. But in my dream, the term called up the image of a dog dripping saliva, morphed into something rabid and ravenous. In my dream, the cancer was both immutable force and immovable object, a lump in Gabe's midsection and an ichor in his blood.

I woke in a sick sweat, still immersed in a dream-sea of pediatric oncologists and chemotherapy. Only people who have lived it, only medical people and those with grave illnesses, can dream of a terminal-illness scenario with so much precision mingled with the surreal, and that precision begets horror. I knew Gabe was safe and pink in his crib, knew that dreams were a tangent to reality, not reality itself. Yet there was a pain in my solar plexus that was insistent, like knowledge. It said: *Love him while you can. He won't be here forever.*

The rhabdomyosarcoma dream was the first to bear that message. There have been others, perhaps five or six of them in all. They've cropped up from time to time throughout his life, usually separated by a sheaf of years. In one, I'm searching for Gabe through a nearly empty hospital ward when I come upon his coffin. That was probably about the time we were out riding the hills so often. In a recent dream that seems like a continuation of that long-ago rhabdo dream, a crucial screening test, due in the spring of 2000, was overlooked; now an unnamed cancer has come back. Gabe is admitted to an oncology unit that is unpopulated and lonely, and his doctor sets about placing a line in a large central vein for chemo. I can see the contents of the central-line kit in my dream, and the square of Tegaderm, a transparent, breathable dressing, that is going to go over the entry site. Gabe's oncologist has a soft air of regret about him. He isn't saying very much. He knows, and I know without being told, that the prognosis is poor. The dream Gabe is frightened. As in waking life, as on the road, Gabe is elaborately casual, but there's a hollowness in his eyes.

And I can't lie to this otherworld Gabe. The specific knowledge of his dream-undoing is in my waking-world fabric. It's in all the coffee I've drunk at two in the morning, sitting outside bone-marrow-transplant rooms. It's in six or seven IV pumps piercing the quiet with their alarms. It's in entering those laminar-flow rooms—after scrubbing, gowning, masking, and gloving—to run ten or twenty potent drugs in the course of a twelve-hour shift into triple-lumen central lines. Lines that belong to kids with cancer, kids who have relapsed once, twice, multiple times after standard treatment. Kids who are bald, pale—refugees from a country no one wants to visit. Hollow-eyed kids. The knowledge is in the smell of vomit, bilious and only faintly acrid when a kid hasn't eaten for weeks, his gut inflamed and eroded from chemo. And it's in the memory of parents sitting next to their kids in the dimness of 2:00 a.m., their yellow gowns blooming like ghosts.

They puzzle me, these dreams. Of course I don't believe in them. They're a symbol of something Freudian, or perhaps they're just an undigested bit of beef, for which I have a fondness, as my cholesterol profile can attest. After all, Gabe is not dead, and his illnesses have been few and slight. I've murmured midnight thoughts with yellow-gowned parents; I know how lucky I really am. Gabe's seventeen now, well over six feet tall. He has grown into his size-fourteen feet. He stops opposing linemen sixty pounds heavier than he is, and once in a while he still finds time to chase around the hills on a bike with me.

Yet I've never dreamed about Kieran this way, not once. Something in me is sure that Kieran will live. Kieran himself, still as enamored of automobiles as he was at three, jokes that he'll probably sail off the edge of a cliff in a favorite car when he's ninety years old. His taste has moved beyond Fords; he sees himself dying at a ripe old age in something sleek and fast. "My grandkids will laugh," he says. "They'll say, 'Yeah, that's Grandpa. At least he went out doing what he loved. But what a shame about that classic Ferrari! He should have left that for us.' "

The truth is that every so often, safe in my own bed in the wee dark hours, Gabe safe in his, I still hear that whisper. *Love him while you can.* It hasn't lost any of its potency.

"I want you to outlive me," I tell him after he's pulled some stunt. This is the closest I can come to it with him. That line has become my shorthand for this prickle of fear that feels so knowing. "I want you to be an old, old man someday. I want you to live long enough to take other kinds of risks. There are intellectual risks, you know. Emotional risks. Like finding out what you're good at, or falling in love."

"Oh, Mom," he says, not without affection. "I understand that you'd miss me and it would be hard for you. But if I die, I'll just be dead. I won't be feeling anything." He wants to roll his eyes, but doesn't. Mostly he's focused on his feeling that his love life, even a potential love life, isn't a topic fit for discussion with his mother. His attention moves off the center of what I'm saying before the words are even out of my mouth. He has millions of fresh new cells thrumming along, murmuring that he's going to live forever. I remember the feeling.

I know I could forbid Gabe's no-handed feats on a bike. He'd grouse, but he'd comply, at least when I was watching. But that's the rub, isn't it? He'd only comply while I was watching, and only with the things I could think of to forbid. Okay, so blasting no-handed down the hill is out, but what about jumping the bike back and forth across the ditch? What about running it full speed down a flight of cement stairs? What about rigging a swing twenty feet up in a tree using frayed rope? I can't forbid him to do things I can't even conceive of. And I can't protect him from the unknowable, from one of his vigorous young cells differentiating in darkness, bent on growing into something that's all wrong.

And finally we're back to the hellraiser in me, who knows it'd be wrong to try. Just yesterday, as I was biking on a quiet street only fifteen minutes into my ride, a car pulled out in front of me. Gabe was at football practice, safe from the *slam-scrape* of the cycling crash, but exposed to the *wham-crush-twist* of the tackle. The car was screened from view until the last possible second by the sweep of the massive cedar that stands sentinel at the verge of driveway and road. I braked too hard; my front wheel slewed sideways on a drift of fallen cedar scales. Body met cracked asphalt. Asphalt produced left-sided road rash, but no loss of consciousness and no fractures, as the trauma nurse in me would report. Just some minor soft-tissue injury.

I accepted Band-Aids from the horrified driver, sat on his stone wall taking deep breaths of slick, rainy air and chatting with him until the shakes subsided. When they stopped, I waved good-bye to my new friend Craig, driver of a white Subaru, husband of a fellow cyclist, and rode on under the evergreens for another forty minutes until fading light forced me home.

There's a silver thread of DNA running through Gabe's cells. It's his mother's half of the helix. It's the hellraiser's, too. It gave him dark curls and introspection, and it gave him a little taste for the edge. He takes it from there. The hellraiser has her own wisdom, which is not the same as the wisdom of a mother. She knows that the heart of where we live is outside our roles as mothers, as sons. She knows there's eternity to be had in a few seconds of speed.

Chapter Seven

A Few Beats of Black Wing

Whtile the fire department extricated our patient from a steaming pile of wreckage a few miles away, my partner and I waited at a baseball diamond in a small-town park hard by the mountains, a grassy expanse scooped out of the dense evergreen of the peninsula. It was a late spring afternoon, hot and dry, and a Little League game was in progress. The game had been suspended while we landed our red-and-white, twin-engine helicopter in a level area of the park; on final approach, the sight of the kids below me, eleven- and twelve-year-old boys from the look of them, made me a little nervous. You can never be sure how well the ground personnel will secure the landing zone, especially in an area like this one, where the fire department is largely volunteer. But the kids had all taken cover in the dugout a good distance away from where we landed, their backs to the dust kicked up by our rotor wash, their hands obediently shielding their eardrums from the roar.

After we shut down and hopped out, the players gawked across the field at the sight of us—royal blue flight suits, steel-toed boots. We pulled off our helmets. My partner was one of my favorite people to work with: smart, funny, the sort of clinician who could size up a situation and do exactly what was necessary, no more, no less. He was tall and muscled, and you'd think he was in his twenties if he didn't have some gray. I was his opposite, short and dark. Ancient pregnancy flab straining the long zipper of my flight suit. We each gave the kids a parade-queen wave. A couple of them waved back.

Eventually a volunteer with a radio informed us it would be a while before our patient arrived. Nothing about it sounded good. Our pilot told the Little League coaches to continue the game until we had to take off again.

Our ground time was more than half an hour, I found later, when I wrote up the flight from the chicken scratches I'd scribbled on two-inch-wide white tape stuck to the Nomex covering my right thigh. A form of eternity. We aim for ten minutes at the most from the time we touch down until the time we lift off again, trying to take advantage of that golden hour after trauma—the brief window in which a patient can be saved if definitive treatment is provided. I kicked at the mown grass as we waited, shrugging my shoulders, watching baseball's small successes—the base hit, the one perfect pitch—and its small defeats—the big whiff, the muffed catch.

We could hear the siren for a couple of minutes before we saw the rig. But at last it kicked up dust in the gravel lot next to the baseball field, its flashing lights washed out in the strong spring sunlight. It was not our first flight of the day, and it was my partner's turn to take report on the patient. Officially, that means he was in charge of the patient's care, though in practice it's almost always collaborative. My turn to package the patient up for transport. He preceded me into the patient bay, taking the big step up through the rig's back door.

It was cooler inside, and dim after the brightness of the afternoon. Backboarded on the stretcher lay a seventeen-year-old boy, a boy the same age as my son was then. He was tall, had straight, dark blond hair. If he was bloody, as he must certainly have been, my memory has filtered that out. I would have expected abrasions and cuts, random splashes of blood, even fractures. I tend to remember only what was striking or pertinent.

CPR was in progress; that was pertinent. The paramedic

held up a hand, signaling the emergency medical technician to stop CPR. I put two fingers at the top of the boy's thigh, in the crease of his groin. With CPR, there had been a faint femoral pulse, which meant compressions were effective. Without it, nothing. And when you took away the electrical/mechanical noise of chest compressions, there wasn't so much as a blip on the monitor. A flat line—asystole.

Asystole in this situation is a death knell. It means the heart is so starved for substrates—blood, oxygen, glucose—that it can't beat, not even a few times a minute. It can't even quiver.

"Head-on collision, estimated speed fifty, medium-sized pickup versus a subcompact, about fifty minutes ago now," the paramedic told us as the EMT resumed compressions. With one hand, he bagged breaths into the boy through an endotracheal tube, and with the other, he shot the contents of an epinephrine syringe, a single dose of a potent cardiac stimulant made for cardiac-arrest situations like this one, into the boy's IV. "Patient was the driver of the subcompact, and it was demolished—on fire department arrival he was half pinned in the car, half on the street. Had a carotid pulse at first, but lost it almost immediately. Pupils initially reactive, now fixed and dilated. We got an IV"—this was no small feat in a patient without a blood pressure who was bleeding out from internal injuries—"and he's had three liters of saline. CPR has been in progress twenty minutes. This is our third milligram of epi," he said, gesturing to the syringe with his chin, "and we've given two milligrams of atropine. There was a fatality in the accident: the driver of the pickup was dead at the scene."

It's gonna be two fatalities, I thought as I worked at putting our equipment on the patient. I knew without asking that my partner was on the same page. He shot me a glance that confirmed my thinking as he listened with a stethoscope to the boy's chest.

"So, good breath sounds bilaterally as you bag him, but

CPR for twenty minutes, three liters of fluid, three doses of epi, pupils fixed and dilated, asystole," he said, summing up. "Do you want us to take him?"

It would have been completely proper, and perhaps easier for the family in the long run, to cease efforts. But the boy was seventeen, and we were out here on a baseball field miles from anywhere with the crack of a bat and the muffled cheers of Little League filtering into the rarefied air of the rig.

"His dad's outside," the medic said, an apparent non sequitur that meant *I think we should try everything.* "He followed us from the scene. His mom works in the city. She's been notified."

He asked the EMT to stop compressions again. "Any response to the epi?"

In the midst of a flat line, a few agonal beats as the epi unsuccessfully flogged a dying heart.

"Well, there you go," the medic said with bright finality, as if a couple of EKG complexes made a difference.

We emerged into dust and sun. My partner took over the airway, squeezed breaths into the patient. Our pilot shouldered our equipment bags and strode over to the helicopter. I wrapped the patient up in our pack, belted him and his IVs down. I grabbed a strap at the corner of the stretcher and lifted, in concert with the EMT and a couple of FD personnel. The medic continued compressions. I was thinking three or four steps ahead. Loading a patient into the helicopter is a kind of dance, choreographed to make sure that everything—everyone—gets stowed, secured, monitored, and that all can communicate. It's dicier when you're breathing for the patient through a tube and when his only circulation comes from hands compressing his breastbone against his heart.

As we made the slow procession to the open door of the aircraft, out of the corner of my eye I saw the boy's dad trailing us. "Hang in there," he kept saying to his son. He was on the verge of crying but managed to hold himself together. "I know you're going to make it. Don't give up."

I've forgotten the boy's name, though his dad called it out, called out to him over and over. Maybe that seems inhuman. It's years ago, many patients ago. Quite a few flights with CPR in progress ago. He was my patient for perhaps forty-five minutes, all told.

What I can say for myself is I remember the solid muscular weight of him as I carried his stretcher, the long elegant lines of his body. He was a caribou, an elk, a gazelle. I remember his hanks of dark blond hair, and I do or do not remember that blood was streaked and caked in it. I remember the resignation of knowing he wasn't going to survive. In its way, it felt as heavy as the stretcher. I thought of my own seventeen-year-old. He was more of a pit bull: short, squat, and ferociously funny. But it was a dry thought and it didn't prod me into feeling anything more. *That dog don't hunt*, I think a southerner might say.

"We're taking him to the trauma center in the city," my partner informed the boy's father.

I know what it's like—how startling it is—to watch a boy shoot up tall in the space of a year, grow biceps and a beard. To hear him drop his new bass-voice concerns into conversation (conversations that can only occur while we're in motion—on walks at night with our faces comfortingly indistinct, on bikes, or behind the wheel as one of us negotiates city traffic) and to hear the unspoken plea *Don't make an overemotional hash of this, Mom!* And I've noticed how a boy's problems transition away from childhood all of a sudden, like the day in late August when the light changes and you know autumn is imminent—*How would you feel if I drank beer at a friend's house with his parents' permission? What exactly is in a mai tai, anyway? I like this girl, she's gorgeous. No, I don't want to tell you her name. I've* retrieved a pack of linemen from football camp, their minds a billion miles away from academics, the windows of the car open to dispel the three-day-old locker-room stench they're so proud of. *Ass, by Calvin Klein,* they joke. I know what it's like to find the Wonderbra Web site up on my computer screen and, later, a franker shade of porn lying out in his room, along with the odd crunchy sock in the laundry. To watch him ratchet the car out of the driveway in reverse at warp speed, a new-minted driver's license steaming in his wallet. A friend and fellow mother of boys, fresh from an inadvertent glimpse of her teenage stepson as he emerged from the shower, mock screamed and said, "No wonder he can't get it together at school. He's growing a dick, and it's all he can do!"

I wanted to tell the dad I'd love his boy as much as I could. But it was already too late. The next hours would be bereft of tenderness, a matter of the process running its course. I opted for busying myself with the stretcher, knowing I was ducking an ill-defined responsibility. Knowing he wasn't ready to hear what I had to say.

The dad picked my brain wave clean out of the air. "Take good care of him," he said. He hurled it like an epithet at my back, a storm edge in his voice.

∞

We had only four hands between us, and they were full. Normally we would have transmitted a short radio report to the trauma center, but instead we asked the pilot to do it: seventeen-year-old male, high-speed head-on MVA, CPR in progress. That was enough, they'd get the idea. Trauma flights from the field—prehospital flights—with CPR in progress end in death almost a hundred percent of the time. If you could scoop a victim out of the wreck and put him directly in the OR with a trauma team standing by, you might sometimes get a save. But not with time and distance working against you, not with miles of sky, an invisible gusher somewhere deep in the interior firmament, and cells winking out by the millions in every body system.

The flight was as most such flights are: more work to do than there are minutes or hands to do it, but with the pressure curiously off. I was out of my seat belt the whole way, half standing in a crouch, half kneeling on the stretcher platform, my butt wedged against the left-side door/window of the cabin so I could get enough leverage to do effective chest compressions. The landscape streaked by below, trees and coves and open water, and over us, the fat fluffy clouds of a hot day in spring. I didn't see any of it. It was about a million degrees in the cabin, and the sweat stung my eyes as the stains under our arms grew. Our little ventilator must have hissed, but we couldn't hear it. I did CPR with my elbow when I needed my hands. My cohort pushed epi every three to five minutes, gave another dose of atropine, and ran in several more liters of fluid—with its general scarcity and its perishability, blood can't routinely be carried, and of course, if the patient needed anything, he needed blood. We never saw a spontaneous pulse or blood pressure. Not a single organized EKG complex. Halfway through the flight, maybe after a dose of epi, a slightly wavy line appeared on the monitor instead of a flat line—a fine ventricular fibrillation. It's not usual or really indicated after trauma, but at that point we had nothing to lose, so we looked at each other, shrugged, and defibrillated him with three stacked shocks, his body convulsing with 200, then 300, then 360 joules of electricity. It didn't change anything.

At the trauma center, the full-court press. Central lines, massive amounts of warmed blood products, his chest cracked open. Everything possible done, yes, and everybody in the room stepping up to practice skills they couldn't acquire in any other situation. Skills that might make the difference on some other patient. The process is as feral as that.

Dozens of people, somebody's hands right on his pale heart. And inevitably, afterward, a ton of garbage on the floor—discarded packaging in paper and plastic, squares of gauze with blood on them, tubes, guide wires—and a single silent house-keeper mopping up.

∽

We were writing our notes at the main desk outside the trauma room, the two of us an island of concentration in the midst of noise and chaos, when the social worker approached us. We were hungry, and tired, and so, so thirsty. I needed a gallon of cold water.

"The mom's out in the waiting room. Would one of you like to talk to her?"

"No," said my partner before she had finished her sentence. It was a peremptory bark, and it startled me. He had a cool elegance under pressure; he was wry and realistic. He'd flown hundreds of hopeless patients like this one. But the afternoon's events had worn on him too, I guess. Abraded him, somehow.

"We have nothing to add," he said. He never looked up from the paperwork.

Ah, but his home is with his much-loved partner of many years. His is a more circumscribed, citified life that includes fresh paint on the walls and a carefully tended garden, parents aging in the Midwest. No children. He doesn't have—can't be expected to have—my uterine understanding of all there is to add. Of how imagination can torture, and how much every de-tail will matter when, her son's body gone to the morgue, that mother drives home to find a grimy school backpack mute in the hall where he dropped it, still stuffed with books, chewed gum, an iPod and earbuds, his crumpled papers.

The social worker turned to walk away. I opened my mouth to say I'd talk to the mom, of course I would. There was nothing I could do about the raw new hole in her family. But I could supply the gap in her knowledge. I knew I could imprint a fellow mother's face on those last-gasp minutes, that final arc of boiling sky between a Little League field and a big-city skyline.

Inside my mental nimbus, where the clatter of the ER couldn't reach, a hummingbird thrummed, a crow flapped a few beats of black wing. I can't say why I didn't speak, only that I wish I had. The social worker's purposeful back disappeared through the double doors that separated the ER from the waiting room; years have passed and I'm still standing there, unable to say a thing.

Chapter Eight

Longview

The temperature's in the mid-eighties, windless, cloudless: a noontime poised at the peak of July perfection, about to clock its descent into the stale nuclear heat of afternoon. We—my sons, Kieran and Gabe, my longtime friend Julie, and I—stand astride our bikes at the on-ramp to the Lewis and Clark Bridge. We're waiting for Seattle-to-Portland (STP) Ride volunteers to stop traffic so hundreds of us on bikes of every description, blazing with every neon color humans can devise, can cross the muddy Columbia River from Washington to Oregon. In the past twenty-eight hours, we've ridden a hundred and fifty miles; fifty miles today, fifty to go to make Portland. We're sweating and saddle sore and stiffening as we wait. Any longer and we'll develop rigor mortis. At this point of the ride, motion is salvation.

Kieran, Gabe, and I have been riding together for three years. We started with a rolling five-mile loop near home, and for the first week or so Kieran and I had to walk up some of the hills. Kieran is eighteen now, going on nineteen, fresh from his first year at Seattle Central Community College. He's moved way beyond our casual tours of the neighborhood; he commutes all over the Seattle area by bike and has been training with a local group of racers for the past year. Gabe and Julie are natural athletes. Gabe's fifteen, going on sixteen, and his main focus is football; his habit for cycling has continued to be a lazy ten miles—*Look, Ma, no hands!*—and only when he feels like it.

Julie is a few years younger than I am. She lives in San Francisco and has flown up for this ride; she's known the boys most or all of their lives. She does not have or want children, but from the first days of our friendship, she always included the boys in our plans. She first met Kieran when he was eighteen months old. I brought him up to the PICU where we both worked and introduced them; he impressed her when he piped up at her from knee height to say, "Let's sit down and have a conversation, Julie!" From then on, she was the one who knew he liked to lunch at the seedy Mission Rock Café on the bay, where he could watch the shipyard across the channel from his high chair. She's a runner and a triathlete; we used to do the 12K Bay-to-Breakers run together in San Francisco, including the year I was twenty-one weeks pregnant with Gabe. As we jogged up the Hayes Street hill that May, right past Julie's apartment at the corner of Alamo Square, we passed a group of runners, immense, struggling linemen from the San Francisco 49ers—fatties, Gabe calls them, now that he's one of them. I marveled at the size (and cellulite) of their thighs.

"Pregnant women are faster than you!" Julie yelled out to them.

Kieran has ridden STP the past two years, but it's the first time for the rest of us. "When they let us onto the bridge," he says now as we wait, seizing up, on the on-ramp, "you've got to pull way out to the left and climb. Just follow me. Go balls-to-the-wall to the top of the span, get ahead of the pack."

Julie snorts and waves him off. "Don't worry about me," she says. "I'm in the mood to take my time."

Gabe stares off into the space above the river, like a cat intent on some phantasm invisible to humans. He gives no sign that he's heard a word his brother has said.

Kieran turns to me. "Don't get boxed in, Mom. That happened to Mike last year, and believe me, it sucked for him."

"Why, exactly, would I want to bust my ass on the bridge?" I ask, and Kieran raises one cocky blond eyebrow.

"Because if there's nobody in front of you, it's *awesome* on the downhill side. I think I hit fifty last year. You'll be *flying* into Oregon."

Mike is one of the guys who races with Kieran. He's my age but whippet-thin, rides a custom titanium Seven that you can lift with a finger, and he can cruise at twenty-five miles an hour. If Mike got boxed in, there's no hope for me.

But I'm still fueled—stoked—by the swift fifty miles we just rode through the soft summer morning, up and over the rollers of southern Washington. Hills so lush and green they were hallucinatory, at least as long as my brain and adrenals and every other imaginable gland pumped out that steady immortal elixir of exercise neurotransmitters. Hills and endogenous chemicals and the most divine double espresso in the world carried me down, down, down the state through Napavine and Winlock, Castle Rock and Lexington, on into Kelso and across Longview's barren miles of cracked industrial asphalt to this small limbo at the foot of the bridge, where the four of us fidget, surprisingly good companions after seventeen years, two complete childhoods, and two descents into middle age.

The bridge pitches toward the sky above us to our right, a mile and a half long, its squat cantilevered midsection suspended 210 feet above the slow roil of the river. When they throw the roadbed open to us, I clip in for the jackrabbit start, hauling hard nose-to-ass with Kieran's baggy, paint-stained gym shorts. He favors the ragamuffin look for casual riding, likes to be the sleeper cyclist, the one whose clothes and weight belie his speed. He weaves me left through the crowd, and I stand up, give it everything I've got—the uphill arc of the bridge is a moderate climb, not nearly as steep as some of the shit I ride at home, and it's *working*, for Christ's sake. Two-thirds of the way up the span, I throw a glance behind me. We've dropped the pack. As we crest over the middle of the Columbia, 210 feet— *ten miles high*—in the clean, cool interstate air, there are only a couple of guys—*Mikes*—in front of us. One of them is Gabe on his mountain bike, pounding out his absentminded, incredibly efficient stroke.

I've crossed the line. Oregon—*the world, the universe*—is laid out below, and I don't brake. Won't. The light-speed sound of the wind—of any wind, of every wind—is roaring in my ears. My sweat has dried, and I know I'm going to live forever. But my sons, heavier, stronger, younger, outdistance me, as they should. As they will. Their two broad backs recede below me, down, down, down around the sweep of cloverleaf and into the workaday traffic of a new state, where I lose sight of them.

Chapter Nine

New Worlds, Like Fractals

1204

It's just four minutes past noon when we climb into the belly of the beast. Tim has the helicopter cranking already. Doreen and I grab our coats and helmets in the hangar, pick up the stock we've laid out ready to put in the bags, and walk across the tarmac at this small suburban airfield.

The airport lies in an unprepossessing valley of farmland and subdivisions, a flat stretch between the cold, deep waters of Puget Sound and the Cascade foothills. There are snowed peaks to the east, a sharp blanket of stars overhead on a fair evening, rain blowing sideways, and, in summer, the loamy stench of fertilizer carried on the evening haze. Today I can't see Mount Baker, a 10,750-footer that sits shivah to the northeast. It's shrouded in clouds that are spitting a little rain, business as usual for autumn in western Washington.

This will be the first flight of our twenty-four-hour shift. The familiar start-up whine of the rotors is just shifting into thunder when Tim gives us the nod that it's safe to approach— the main rotor can flex down to decapitation height at slow speeds. Doreen heads around the nose of the helicopter to the right-side seat, behind the pilot. I duck under the rotors to the left, slide in. The left side is the airway-management side— if our patient needs to be intubated, I'll have the best ergonomics. And if something ugly happens to both our engines, if we go down in the sound, Tim's probably going to roll it to my side as we hit. Thanks, Tim. I'll be the one underwater, dodging the blades, if I'm not pulverized by the impact first.

But I don't waste time worrying about that—I love it more than a little. As the engines rev, it's the sound: the outsize roar, the prickle of fear and the surge of exhilaration, the way the aircraft vibrates until it's running at full speed, ready for takeoff. The shimmy reminds me I'm buckling myself in to the eye of a maelstrom. True, it's a tight ship of a maelstrom, controlled in our 1983 Agusta by the laws of physics, our pilot with his thousands of hours of military and commercial flying, and clever but aging feats of engineering. The potential for havoc thrums away somewhere unseen, somewhere like my bone marrow, largely unacknowledged. But all three of us, I'm pretty sure, get the same kick out of the moment of lift, when the earth slips off our shoulders and we climb, nose down, toward the sun. I use the term *sun* loosely.

Tim radios dispatch, calls us off at 1211 with an ETA of about twelve minutes to the rooftop helipad of the referring facility, a small hospital on the coast of the Olympic Peninsula. Armand, in dispatch, gives us the short report: we're going for a sixty-one-year-old male with a heart attack—an inferior myocardial infarction. The small hospital does not have a cardiac catheterization lab; they can't open up his clotted, blocked coronary arteries there. And time means heart muscle dying from lack of blood flow; that's why we're flying him.

His destination, the receiving hospital, is unusual, a first for this kind of flight. Instead of going to one of the big cardiac centers in Seattle, we're taking him to a medium-sized suburban hospital about thirty-five miles away. We go to this particular hospital all the time, but to transport patients out. They don't have a neurosurgeon on staff, and they often call us for intracranial bleeding: head injuries and strokes. On one memorable Sunday, I flew four patients to Seattle from there, possibly a record for most flights in one day from the same facility. But their cardiac catheterization lab is brand-new; it's the first time in my experience that they'll be receiving a patient.

Five months ago, my mother was admitted to this same receiving hospital, ratcheted over fifteen miles of freeway black-top under lights and sirens. The reason: an inferior MI. But right now I am so dialed in to my work mode that these facts don't raise a blip on my internal radar. Nor do I remember that she and my father lived for several years in a retirees' apartment, practically under the shadow of the sending hospital, in the same small coastal town. That sort of private information is stowed in some other set of brain cells, on a different circuit.

I glance over at Doreen; she comes to flight nursing from a background in adult critical care. I'm experienced in the maternal/child specialties—obstetrics, pediatric and neonatal ICU. She smiles and nods. She'll take report on this patient, will direct his care, and I'll package him up to fly. She's fairly new, but I love working with her—she's calm, sweet but smart, has a quirky Canadian sense of humor. Between the two of us, things tend to stay loose. I pull my little reference book out of the flight-suit pocket down by my right ankle and jot down some drug doses on a two-inch-wide strip of white tape I've stuck onto my thigh—IV nitroglycerin, a few different classes of anticoagulants. I don't know what he's on or what we'll need to start. I know the dose ranges fairly well, but adult cardiac care isn't my strong suit, and it's kind of a Zen thing for me to write them down. If our guy develops some unusual, unfriendly cardiac rhythm, I'll be looking to Doreen to boss me around. As we lift, I strap the IV pump to the stretcher with the bags. Everything's as ready as it can be.

Cornfields, the Safeway plaza, Interstate 5, tract developments, and after a few minutes, the fragile white backbone of the shoreline slide by underneath us as we head west toward the white mass of the Olympic Mountains. We're cruising at about fifteen hundred feet, and the November afternoon is chilly in our little bubble of a cabin. The heater is almost painfully loud, white noise in big decibels, and most of the time we do without it. The patients are wrapped up like burritos in several layers, one of which is a space blanket. They're never cold unless they're in shock from blood loss, trauma, or infection. The three of us just hunker into our jackets and down vests.

The sound is an ashen gray today, reflecting the sky, rippled with waves that are probably quite large to the small boats flecking the surface down there. Tim talks to Paine Field tower on the radio as we fly through their airspace; we make a little small talk over the intercom when there's no radio traffic. Doreen, who's single, is going home to her parents' place for Thanksgiving. I mention that it's my oldest son's birthday tomorrow—he'll be seventeen. I say I hope we don't fly all night, because when quitting time comes at 0900, 9:00 a.m., tomorrow, I'll have to shop for a birthday present and a cake.

For his birthday, Kieran wants ultralight, exotic (expensive!) racing wheels for his Cannondale, or rollers that will force him to balance in place while he trains for two hours a night watching episodes of *Friends*. He's five-eight, and before he started biking, he weighed 320 pounds, 120 pounds more than his current weight. I can't quite afford racing wheels but am thinking they might be considered propitiation to the gods of weight loss. I'm proud of Kieran and relieved, impressed by the new adult grit he's shown, finding his own way to battle biochemistry and genetics on that front.

As we sweep across the sound, the plume of steam from the paper mill in our destination town comes into view. Tim circles once around the hospital, the local houses and the ocean changing places at a kaleidoscopic cant. The lost seventh-grader in me, the one who could eat three questionable corn dogs for lunch and ride the roller coaster all afternoon, grooves on it for a second. Before nausea can set in, Tim sets us down gently on the tiny pad, inside the crosshairs painted onto the roof.

∞

MONDAY, JUNE 3, 6:00 P.M.

My dad called me around six in the evening. "Your mother's having trouble catching her breath," he said.

"How long has this been going on?" I asked Dad.

"Since about noon," he said. "But it's getting worse."

Mom was legally blind as well as walker/wheelchair–dependent from complications of diabetes. She was also on hemodialysis three times a week and had been dialyzed last on Saturday. My dad took care of her at home, but he hated dealing with her medical issues. He didn't trust doctors or the health-care juggernaut.

"Here, talk to her," he said. I could practically see him shoving the receiver at her. *Take this cup from me*, I thought randomly.

The past few months had been difficult for Mom. She wasn't sleeping at night, complaining of heartburn, and I had been wondering if it was really angina, not heartburn. She kept my father awake too, and he had lost weight, was exhausted, looked pale and anorexic.

She'd had hallucinations: children in white playing in the yard, coming up to press their faces against the door. All spring, I had the feeling of an ill wind blowing.

"Hey, Mom," I said. "How are you doing?"

I had seen them both the previous Thursday evening, at the middle school spring band concert. Gabe played the flute at a school with a good music program, and my mother never missed a performance. "I love that huge sound pouring over me," she'd said, her wheelchair planted firmly in a prime spot. Never the back wall for *my* mother. She was strictly front row. And at every seasonal concert she said the same thing: "They play so well! The band teacher is doing a marvelous job with those kids."

My parents were themselves retired professional musicians. My mother was a pianist and organist, my father a choir director and choral conductor; but both of them were singers straight from the bel canto tradition, and singing was what they loved. My mother was a soprano. In the 1950s, she had attended the Boston Conservatory but left to study in New York with bel canto vocal coach Enrico Rosati. Mario Lanza was also one of his students.

For most of their working lives, before they retired out west, my parents were music directors at Boston-area Catholic parishes large enough to support serious music programs. Throughout my childhood, I'd sung in their choirs. The whole family had. We could sing in four parts, just the seven of us. Mom, Christine, and I were sopranos, Bernadette and Camille were altos, my father was the tenor section, and once Kevin's voice changed, he became our bass.

All her life, Mom's voice had been her instrument. In her prime, it was a huge voice—the sort that penetrates bone and muscle, pierces emotional ice and melts it. A voice that was made for the passion and pathos of Puccini, or for entreaties to heaven. Sometimes against my will, it had brought tears to my eyes when she was in her sixties. And even at seventy-two, after fifteen years of poorly controlled diabetes and its devastating inroads, her voice still had great vibrancy and timbre, all the vigor of the lusty Italians she descended from. It *carried*.

But not that night, not on the phone. "Not doing so good," she was saying, and I could barely hear her. What I did hear clearly was the wheezy hitch between each word as she fought for air.

"Let me speak to Dad again," I said.

"I think you need to call nine-one-one," I told him when he came back on the line. "I can come over, but it'll take me forty-five minutes. A waste of time. The medics can do a few things to help her breathe, and they'll take her to the hospital. I can meet you there."

I wondered, on my thirty-mile drive down to the hospital, if she had gone and done it this time. She'd had a lot of close calls before, but she'd always managed to regain some equilibrium, just enough health to come home and keep going. Enough for her to stay on the other end of the phone when I called, come out to lunch with me every few weeks, bedevil me about ghosts and levitation. She had a lifelong interest in the paranormal. We all did.

I think I knew what was coming. The drive down felt like the last outpost of an old life.

There was a medic unit on the ramp outside the ER; I knew, by the city and unit number, that it had to be hers. Obeying the rules, I went through the patients' entrance, inquired for her at the triage desk. My work self, the self who knew the code to the ambulance door, was the one in some other compartment. The triage nurse waved me through.

Inside the big room, all five curtained spaces were full. I found her intubated and on a ventilator, a paramedic next to her gurney. He was finished with his paperwork, just about to depart.

"I'm Greg," he said, shaking my hand. "I transported your mom."

He was middle-aged—salt-and-pepper hair, short and wiry. Kind blue eyes. And I recognized him. Years before, on my third flight ever, I had picked up a teenager from him, a female with chest injuries from a head-on motor vehicle crash on a nearby highway. As I packaged her in the back of his rig, I found that the regulator for our oxygen tank was broken. I was new and overwhelmed, and a broken regulator seemed like a professional gaffe, a mini-tragedy. But he quietly lent me one, and he was courteous about it, no carping about where and how he would get it back. People are protective of their equipment out there—it's expensive. Since I live only five or six miles from his fire station, I was able to promise to return it personally.

He didn't seem to remember me, however, and I wanted the professional story, not the simplified version most people get.

"I'm Jennifer," I said. "I'm one of the flight nurses, by the way. How'd it go?"

"Well, she was short of breath. It was a little better when I sat her up. We started her IV at the house and loaded her into the rig, but we no sooner got around the corner when she got worse, more panicky and agitated. She kept saying, 'I can't breathe.' She didn't sound wet, particularly, but her oxygen saturations were dropping a bit and it was clear she needed some help. So I put her down with etomidate and succinylcholine, and intubated her with a seven-point-five tube. It went well, her sats came up, she was easy to bag, and we got here, no problem. She had a stable blood pressure throughout."

"Yeah," I said. "When I heard her on the phone this afternoon, I was thinking she might need to be tubed. Thanks for taking such good care of her. I appreciate it."

"Hope she does well. I understand she's on dialysis? We saw her central line. We didn't use it."

"Yeah. I hope she just got a little fluid overloaded, but I don't know. I wonder if she might not be having an MI. Did you guys do an EKG?"

"Yup. Nothing leaped out at me. These folks"—he indicated the gaggle of people at the ER desk—"have it."

Then I was alone with her for the moment, alone in the bright hubbub of the ER, and I took stock. Her blood pressures were a little high; hypertension was one of her chronic problems. The thing that made me grit my teeth was that she was starting to wake up—gagging a bit on the endotracheal tube, her eyes opening from time to time, streaming tears. Not with-it enough to try and talk yet, to find out that the tube prevents talking. But close. And despite several surgeries and two years of dialysis, or maybe because of them, she had a frank dread of all things medical.

She wasn't a calm person by nature. She was as operatic as her voice, for one thing, a diva who thought nothing of pointing a blunt, stubby finger to the menial tasks she expected her minions—husband, children, grandchildren—to perform for her. She could flare with the kind of anger that once prompted her to flush an entire meal of veal parmigiana down the toilet after her own father criticized her cooking. Anger with an eye for a flourish, a huge appetite for fun never far offstage. And there was an edge of anxiety beneath her bluster that also softened any impatience I might have had with her. She projected, sometimes, the terror of a four-year-old lying awake in a dark bedroom. Grand sense of humor, stage left. In the wings, unseen monsters, biding their time.

∞

1227

I'm glad it's afternoon and not three in the morning, when energy ebbs to its most negligible. For a cardiac flight, we have to schlep everything—stretcher, monitor, defibrillator, both bags, the IV pump. It adds up to a lot of weight to balance and carry, and a lot of equipment to keep track of. On other types of calls, on a scene call for trauma, for example, we can leave most of it behind in the helicopter.

We trundle down to the ER and I hang a left into a small exam room where we find the gentleman we are to transport. He is pleasant, cooperative, weighs about a hundred kilos, has received morphine, and is on IV nitroglycerin for chest pain. He currently rates his pain as a 2 on a scale of 0 (meaning no pain) to 10 (the greatest pain imaginable). We'll continue to address the pain issue; even a little pain equals dying heart muscle. I give him a few more milligrams of morphine, plan to increase his nitroglycerin next if the pain doesn't abate. I tell him what the weather is like, what the helicopter is like inside, how I think the flight will go, and how long it will take. Tim comes into the room, bringing his large, somewhat alpha-male presence with him, and the patient is obviously, even a little pathetically, relieved to meet him. Perhaps he was afraid *I* was the one who was going to fly the thing. I give Tim a Hollywood buildup, tell the patient that he's the best pilot on earth. And he is, even if his emergency plan does include rolling me into the freezing Puget Sound.

Our guy is able to joke with me and with Tim a little, and I decide he isn't overly anxious about flying, not he-needs-Valium anxious. While I switch his medications over to my IV tubing and pump, I give him the spiel about chest pain and heart muscle, how our goal is zero pain, and stoicism isn't in his own best interest. Many people, and especially men, lie to us about their pain, feel it's somehow important to gut it out. Sometimes they'll lie to us even after the spiel. They'll risk worse damage to their hearts rather than say, "I hurt."

They're being dense. It's frustrating to me as a care provider, but my heart goes out to them a little. There's something in it I recognize. The human capacity for resilience and for accommodation to conditions continually amazes me. And we all have such a need for normalcy. If we have to, we'll pretend we're okay while the elephant sits on our chests—pales our faces, beads sweat on our foreheads, raises our heart rates, forces out those soft, involuntary moans. If we have to, we'll pretend that it's just an everyday thing, like doing the vacuuming, when we pack up people who are critically ill, load them into roaring tin cans, and lift them into the air.

In other news, our patient has a heart rhythm that's a little slow—I'm guessing he received a beta-blocker, a drug that takes some of the strain off his heart. It decreases the heart rate. He's got a good blood pressure, so I'm not worried about it. His EKG, sitting on the bedside table, shows the changes I'd expect to see with an inferior MI. He got an aspirin in the field from the paramedics, and he's on appropriate doses of a couple of other IV drugs—those drugs I wrote down on my right thigh—that will also prevent further clotting. He tells me he doesn't have any drug allergies or a history of problems that might cause catastrophic bleeding, like a hemorrhagic stroke or recent surgery, now that he's so nicely anticoagulated. He hasn't taken any Viagra in the past couple of days either, at least not that he's willing to mention to me. Drugs for erectile dysfunction taken together with nitroglycerin can significantly decrease blood pressure.

My partner comes in from talking to the ER doc, takes a listen to our patient's chest, tells me he sounds clear. That's good: fluid isn't backing up into his lungs from a failing heart. We move him over to our stretcher, bundle him up in our bright yellow burn pack (the reason we call it a burn pack is lost somewhere in the mists of our organizational history). I try to secure the IV bags and pump so the pump won't suck air into its tubing, a problem that's a headache to fix and denies the patient his medications while I purge his lines. I heft one medical bag and the patient's belongings. Tim carries the other bag and the defibrillator. Doreen has the paperwork and pushes the gurney with our stretcher (and the patient) on it. Our guy says he's a little too warm, and we tell him we'll loosen things up for him in the helicopter if he still feels that way once we're out in today's gray chill. We troop up to the roof, and as soon as the door opens, a freshening wind blasts at us from the southwest.

"I'm not hot anymore," the patient pipes up. "But that wind sure feels good. For a while I was wondering if I'd ever feel it again."

"Hey, you've got a lot of living left to do, my friend," says Doreen.

After we grunt and shoehorn the guy's hundred kilos into the cabin and stow all our gear, Tim fires up the aircraft, lifts us straight off the pad, points us southeast. It'll be about a fifteen-minute flight.

∞

MONDAY, JUNE 3, 8:00 P.M.

Mom's heart rate was 140, fast and panicky. If she was having an MI, her heart was working way too hard.

Not enough sedation, I said to myself. I almost reached down to pull narcotics out of the leg pocket of my nonexistent flight suit.

The ER doc stopped by the bedside, and I mentioned my concerns about how awake she was. I know some of the ER physicians by sight, but he was unfamiliar. He was busy—evening shift always is—and harried.

"She's had two milligrams of Ativan," he said, a little aggrieved.

Whoopee ding-dong, the four-year-old in me felt like replying. But instead I pointed out the heart rate of 140, the tears on her cheeks. "It doesn't seem to be doing the trick," I said.

I knew I was walking a tightrope. I needed to stick up for her, and I know more about medicine than most patients and family members. I can't pretend I'm somebody else. But it's so easy to cross that invisible line, turn into a liability: the "difficult" family member. It happens in a flash. It'd be my karmic comeuppance, actually—I've rolled my own eyes way more than once in the past thirty years after turning away from a complaining patient or family member. Medicine is business and time management, as well as science and empathy. Medicine is a whole unit full of sick patients, not just one.

The ER doc told me that her kidney specialist, who also acted as her primary care doctor, was on his way in. And he grudgingly wrote an order for two more milligrams of Ativan, which was a start, though I didn't think in the big picture that it would be enough. I didn't look forward to pestering him for more. He disappeared before I could ask him about her EKG, discuss the potential causes for what had happened.

My white-haired dad came in for a couple of minutes. He had huge bruised bags under his eyes, and I hadn't noticed before how much his pants hung on him. The belt was all that was holding them up—he wouldn't tip the scale at 120 pounds. He used to be nearly six feet tall, but age and arthritis had shrunk him. He leaned, exhausted, on the gurney rail. He didn't touch my mother, could barely bring himself to look at her.

"The poor darlin'," he said, gesturing toward her. "What do you think?"

"I don't know, Dad. Did she complain of chest pain or heartburn today?"

"Not today," he said. "You know I'm always feeding her Tums, and lately it's been bad at night, but at about noon she just started saying it was hard to breathe."

"Did she drink a lot of fluid this weekend? More than usual?"

"No. I don't think so. That was one thing she was always pretty careful about."

There was a silence. "Why don't you go home, Dad?" I said finally. "I'm sure they'll be keeping her here, and I can stay until things get sorted out for the night. You look like you need to get some sleep."

He was dying to get out of there; all he needed was permission. He couldn't stand the blinding, mechanized hum of the place, the tube in her mouth, and the thought of dealing with doctors. He was just holding on with his fingernails. Taking care of her was too much, was killing him, in fact. I had tried, in the past, to set up housekeeping help, nursing help. But between the two of them, they'd nixed every plan.

"It doesn't do any good," he'd say. "It's not what I need."

"Your father can do all that," she'd say, waving a hand. "We want our privacy."

They lived with my sister Bernadette and her family, in a basement studio apartment, and Bernadette had offered to do Mom's shower twice a week. It was a bit of a production because Mom wasn't very mobile and had a big IV line with two ports for dialysis that needed to be protected from water. But whenever Bernadette came at the appointed time to do the shower, Mom would have some excuse for why it wasn't the right moment. Or no excuse—"I just don't feel like it right now!" she'd snap, pouting. What she really wanted was for my dad to do it. She felt he owed it to her, somehow.

And what Dad really wanted was for us, his children, to take care of her. She had been sliding downhill for more than seven years, and we pitched in wherever we could. But there was an unbridgeable gap between their expectations and what we could realistically do. I had always thought I'd walk through fire for those I love, move any mountain, but my time flutters away like confetti on the wind, my loyalties divided. The huge reservoir of energy I had at twenty has evaporated. And something happened that I hadn't expected. Caring has acquired a patina of guilt, and fury. The need is bottomless, and I can't meet it.

A few minutes after Dad left, Mom's nephrologist parted the curtain and entered our flimsy sanctum. I had accompanied my mom to most of her office appointments; I knew him pretty well. He's a silver-haired guy, expensively dressed under his lab coat. He's good at what he does, had always responded to my mother's needs; had, in fact, kept her alive with dialysis for the past two years. He exudes the business sense that enabled him to start his own dialysis center.

He's not exactly warm, though, and my mother sometimes made fun of him over lunch after an office visit. She would sit in her wheelchair at the Olive Garden, her posture erect, eccentric, and dignified in a bright red winter coat that I could never persuade her to take off. She'd splatter things on it as she ate, but her eyesight was practically nonexistent; she couldn't see the small crusts of dried sauce on her lapels. There was no way to keep that coat completely clean. We settled for scraping it off once in a while.

"He just lifts up my shirt and hefts my stomach in his hands," she'd say, imitating it with big Italian gestures and laughing. "What's he feeling around for down there? And he doesn't say so much as 'Please'! No siree, he just lifts up my shirt. What kind of a bedside manner is that? How would he like it if I did that to him?"

"I think he's trying to tell if there's fluid in there or just fat," I couldn't help saying. "But you're right, though, Mom. He's smart, but a bit short on the niceties sometimes."

With me, he was a little judgmental. He was yet another person with firm ideas about how much I should be doing for my mother, ideas that didn't correspond to the tempo of my life, or my other responsibilities—sons, husband, home. Job. Nor did they correspond to the reality of her personality. On one visit, he was upset that she didn't check her blood sugar as much as she was supposed to. "*You* should make sure that happens," he'd said to me.

I was taken aback. "I can't *make* her do it," I'd said. "I know it's a shock, but she doesn't always listen to me. And I can't be over there every day handing her the glucose meter."

"Oh, now, don't tell me that," he had admonished. He actually wagged a finger in my direction. I'd resisted an urge to bite it. Did he think we women were still wearing kerchiefs, meeting at the well in the village square? Preparing breakfast and lunch for the menfolk when they came in from the fields? There seemed to be a world of presumption there, so out of place it almost made me laugh. I wanted to ask him how free *he* was to personally oversee every aspect of his own mother's care.

But that evening in the ER, he shook my hand, and I was glad to see him. "Hey," he said, "what's all this about?"

"I was going to ask you the same question. You heard the story?"

"They called and filled me in when she arrived here in the ER. You know it's been more than two days since she was last dialyzed. Probably she just drank a little too much this weekend and has some fluid in her lungs. We'll dialyze her, and that'll take care of things."

"Well, I hope that's it. But according to my father, she hasn't had more to drink this weekend than any other weekend. After two years, why would she do this all of a sudden?" I asked. "I'm a little concerned that she's having an MI."

He stared at me as if I had three heads. "She didn't complain of chest pain today."

"No, she didn't. But there are her complaints of heartburn, and then again, she's an elderly female with long-standing diabetes." Diabetes damages the nerves that carry pain signals, and women are more likely than men to have atypical symptoms of a heart attack. Of course, he must have known that. I was pushing into pain-in-the-ass territory again, I could tell, and of course I might have been totally wrong about the whole thing, but I pressed on anyway. I felt that at the very least, I should advocate for my mother as well as I do for belligerent drunks I'll never see again.

"She fits the profile of someone who might not present with chest pain. How does her EKG look?" I asked.

"Nonspecific changes," he said. "They've drawn some cardiac enzymes, but there aren't any results yet." Cardiac enzymes are blood tests that look for the by-products of heart-muscle damage.

"How about her chest x-ray? Does it look wet?"

He moved his hand back and forth, an equivocal motion.

"We'll start with dialysis; she'll need that regardless," he said. "We'll admit her to the ICU. Hopefully we can get some fluid off and extubate her in a day or two."

"Okay. And how about sedation? Ativan isn't cutting it." She was still restless, mouthing the tube. Still tachycardic to the 130s. The tears staining her cheeks were getting under my skin.

"We'll put her on a propofol drip once she gets to the ICU."

I had to persist. "And how about now?" I asked. "I know it'll take them a while to get her over there and set it up." Hours, in fact. Propofol is a continuous drip, an IV anesthetic with a short half-life that is used for sedation in the ICU setting.

I could see that at least a part of him wanted to roll his eyes. But professional restraint prevailed, and he jotted down the order for some other drugs.

∞

1255

The flight itself is anticlimactic, as are 95 percent of our flights. We've done all the work already unless our guy pulls something funky, and he doesn't. We start our charting, but the flight is too short to complete it. Blood pressures cycle automatically every five minutes. We both keep an eye on his rhythm and rate. It bumps along between 58 and 64. Doreen radios the patient's status to our medical control in Seattle, who promises to call the receiving hospital with an update, and we learn that we are to proceed directly to the cath lab on arrival—they're ready for us.

Periodically I lean forward to our patient's left ear, lift his earmuff, ask if he has any pain; he denies any. I have to strain to hear his answer over the roar of the engines. I'm seated behind and to the left of him, and what I can see of him—his left shoulder and ear, his left eyeglass frame and cheek (admittedly not a representative sampling)—looks comfortable enough. He is sitting up at about a thirty-degree angle, a little oxygen blowing through his nasal cannula. He feels well enough to turn his head, to take in the view. I wonder what he thinks of it. The world, to my eye, is so vulnerable down there. Ships are tiny, like bathtub models a two-year-old could break, and the sound is a flat slate with baby waves, its boundaries—its limitations—clear. I could blink and miss the Hood Canal Bridge, threading the water between the mounded evergreens of Jefferson and Kitsap counties. Only the Olympic Mountains have heft or weight, and they're behind us.

Tim puts us down in our usual landing zone, a cracked asphalt patch behind a middle school a few blocks from the receiving hospital. Our guy is doing fine, and an ambulance runs all four of us to the ER.

There are two doors side by side on the ER ramp, separate entrances for ambulances and for patients. The patients' entrance catches my eye as I hop out of the back of the rig. And it's right then, between two compartmentalized sets of brain cells, professional and private, that the arc is made.

∞

TUESDAY, JUNE 4, 12:01 A.M.

Just after I helped transfer Mom from the ER gurney into the ICU bed, her nurse told me her cardiac enzymes had come back positive.

"It looks like she's had an MI," the nurse said as she primed tubing with milky, lipid-based propofol. The nurse didn't know I had been worried about that possibility all evening. I looked up at the monitor, where my mom's heart rate was still a rapid, oxygen-guzzling 125, her blood pressure hanging somewhere like 160/90.

"I'm going to give her some metoprolol to decrease the workload on her heart," she said. "It's a beta-blocker."

Yeah. The five or six hours her heart had already hammered along without help weighed on me. I tasted bitterness at the back of my throat.

What now? I asked myself after the nurse had left. It was past midnight, and the room was dark except for the blinking lights of the equipment—monitor, pumps, ventilator. The ventilator whished twelve times a minute, rhythmic and lulling, and my mom's chest rose and fell along with it. With the metoprolol, her heart rate came down to 80.

For most of my adult life, the ICU room, especially at night, has been a comforting place—dim, ordered, and peaceful. It's a weird peace, admittedly, achieved by technology and drugs. But underneath the technologic clutter there *is* a sense of healing taking place. Of buying people time with technology while their tissues mend, while their immune systems get to work. And for the people staffing the ICU, the wee hours of a quiet night can induce a kind of soporific calm. You multitask all evening to make some order out of chaos. You're on your feet for hours, busy every second, to ensure that your patients are assessed, safe, clean, and tolerably comfortable. That you've picked up on all the problems and dealt with them while their doctors are still awake. You make sure that your patients' treatments have been optimized to the extent that it's in your power to optimize them.

In the wee hours of the morning comes your payoff, if you're lucky. You sit in a rocker, write down numbers on a huge flow sheet or click them into a computer once an hour, give some IV medications, maybe siphon some labs once in a while from an arterial line and deal with the results. You talk to your friends. There is a pull toward sleep, but after years on nights some group of cells deep in your brain knows that sleep is off-limits. The peeping of the equipment is soft, hypnotic. Your mind floats a bit. The night, limitless, presses against the windows, kept at bay.

Propofol works fast, and my mother was finally drugged enough to imitate a peaceful sleep. The sheets were clean. She looked warm, tucked in. I put my hand on her forehead, the way she used to feel mine for fever when I was little. It was finally free of the disoriented, half-conscious furrows that I had been trying to smooth away all evening.

The quiet room lulled me. But this was my mother. I didn't know what I should feel, but I didn't think a sense of well-being quite fit the circumstances. I wondered, not for the first time, how much normal human feeling and decency my career had cost me. But I'm not sure the answer is even relevant. And anyway, I knew the calm would last only until the hemodialysis nurse arrived. He would flip on all the lights, make a ruckus setting up equipment.

It's vertiginous, the way parent-child roles reverse. It's no less dizzying because it happens over a period of years, as organs and limbs fail, as brain cells die, as energy fades. Standing next to my mother's bed, I could feel the shadow of my own decline from formless years ahead, reaching toward me like the leading edge of a storm system. Could see some outline of the decisions that Kieran and Gabe, someday, might have to make on my behalf.

Nobody was rushing in to suggest cardiac catheterization or surgery, which I assumed would involve a flight to another center with my compadres. Nobody mentioned treatment to open up her blocked coronary arteries at all. It was as if the possibility wasn't even on the table, or maybe it was just that it was a community hospital, after all, and the decision-makers, her doctors, had gone home. It was a little late in the game, I thought, for thrombolytics, clot-buster drugs like TPA. Her symptoms had been going on for more than twelve hours; the drugs' efficacy declines after a while.

I had a choice to make. I had to decide whether to blow a whistle, make a stink, get doctors on the phone and the helicopter in the air. Whether to rustle her like a shanghaied steer from this quiet oasis out into the cool June night, to the whine and roar of the aircraft. To hustle her off to scalpels and needles, to the brightly lit, brutal uncertainties of an urban cardiac center.

I had tried to discuss end-of-life issues with my mom more than once, usually in the car on our way to some medical appointment. It was maddening and fruitless. I don't think she herself knew what she wanted. She had no idea what was involved in end-of-life heroics, and I couldn't raise her consciousness. She'd shudder and tune out whenever I started to describe things like intubation and CPR, or the vast, slippery slope of a continuum that runs from recovery to hopelessness.

"Well, when I go, I go!" she'd say brightly, her face set against me. "When I kick the bucket, that'll be it for me." Every conversation on the subject came down to those two statements. They were her mantras.

What about disability? I always wanted to scream. It's not like we're guaranteed life—healthy, happy life—to be followed immediately (and conveniently) by the big chill. But then I'd really *see* her: weak, blind, in pain from diabetic neuropathy, needing me to lift her into and out of the car, buckle her seat belt, manhandle the wheelchair. I'd watch her fumble to give herself insulin that somebody else had to draw up, muff her repeated attempts to work the window button in my car. My father helped her dress at four in the morning three times a week so she could travel to the dialysis center in the wheelchair van, so she could sit in the chair for four or five hours, dizzy whenever her blood pressure dipped, as her dark venous blood ran through the dialyzer over and over. It was a process that took nearly nine hours, door to door. I'd try to talk her through the episodes of confusion that were beginning to happen more often; would listen, troubled, as she talked about the vaporous children in white who pressed their noses to the door, who hid in the corners of her apartment. She didn't need *me* to tell her about disability.

The one thing she was clear on was that she didn't want to be cremated.

"Oh, no. I know it's a little stupid, dear, but I'm afraid I'll still be alive when they put me in the fire," she had said, laughing at herself a little, getting me to laugh with her. "I'll wake up in that pine box, smell smoke . . . no, no. That's not for me."

None of this was helping me, there by her bedside. By rights, it was my father's decision, but I knew he didn't want to make it. Officially, there wasn't even a decision to make. The option for some sort of revascularization strategy hadn't been offered by her doctors. I was operating solely off my own experience, and I'm no goddess of cardiology, that's for sure.

The pumps and monitor blinked and clicked. I thought about how much damage her heart muscle was likely to have sustained since she'd started having trouble breathing, an overt sign of congestive heart failure. About whether, if she had extensive, permanent myocardial damage, rehab was likely, given her big list of problems and her passivity about her heath. My mom was the sort of person who lived in the moment. She was never one to look down the gun barrel of the years, envision what was ahead. She didn't believe that today's actions would change the face of tomorrow. Not one whit, really.

Diabetes had trashed her, in large part because she had ignored it for so many years. It doesn't hurt while it's doing its work, undermining nerves, laying gunk down in blood vessels. It's easy to ignore. She had a big appetite, a drive to eat. Obesity wounded her all her life. Her mark of Cain.

She never found a way to get on the right side of her own metabolism, and certainly the medical establishment had no real answers for her. I share her genes, and have fought the same battles with weight and food, but my skinny father and his skinny Irish female relatives also figure in my mix, and I don't believe my struggle has been as desperate. It's Kieran who understands her best: the minute-to-minute metabolic ups and downs, the hunger and cravings that will not be ignored, the way fat can seem like a living thing with its own agenda.

I thought about all the episodes of "heartburn" Mom had been having for the past months, her sleeplessness, my father's gaunt, haunted look. I thought about life in a nursing home, among the strangers she didn't even want in her apartment for a few hours a week. I considered what might have happened if we hadn't called 911, set the emergency medical machinery in motion.

The dialysis nurse arrived and began to set up. The lights were on. He was deft, meticulous, intelligent. And he had been a competitive cyclist who had done very well in national time trials, as we would find out in the coming days. He would talk bikes with Kieran over my mom's still, drugged form.

"I know Jo from the dialysis center," he confided to me. "We're old friends. I'll be able to get some fluid off her, make this better."

I kissed her moist forehead, murmured that I loved her, felt the weight of the world.

"Derek," I said. "I know you'll take good care of her. I'll be back in the morning."

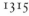

1315

They're ready for us in the cath lab. It's a clean, high-tech room with imaging and monitoring equipment, and a table in the center. Together with the staff, Doreen and I transfer our pleasant sixty-one-year-old gentleman onto the table, instructing him not to struggle to help, to let us do the work. The cath lab has a slide board—a smooth plastic sheet that allows for a controlled *whump* onto the narrow table. He's centered perfectly, a minor miracle.

He blinks behind his thick glasses, courtly and quiet. I can feel his apprehension, but his chest pain must have been very bad at home. He's a little afraid, but also resigned. Ready to move forward to whatever fate awaits him. It's a form of courage, that willingness to face facts.

I feel something large for him in that instant, even though I'll never see him again. For a second, I envision an airy room, filled with imperfect, watery sunlight—a room of this world, not the next. I wish him forward, into it, even as I begin to feel the usual relief that he is no longer my responsibility, start looking forward to a peaceful flight over the countryside, to my lunch back at quarters. A cheeseburger, it'll be, loaded with fat and cholesterol. I won't have any problem handling the irony.

I tell the staff what his IV medications are, leave them running into him on my pump while they set up their own drips. I make the mental note to retrieve the pump before we leave; it's very easy to forget it, fly off and leave it forty-five miles behind me. Doreen is ready to give report. I gather the rest of our equipment, pull our stretcher out into the hallway. I make up the burn pack with clean sheets, fold it lengthwise in thirds, and belt down our bags on top of it, snug and secure.

Back inside the lab, the cardiologist comes toward us. He's bespectacled and middle-aged, exudes a competent, collegial friendliness.

"Wow, you guys made great time," he says. "But we're ready for you."

I should have anticipated him, but I didn't. I wonder if he remembers me from last June. It's eons ago, in medical time, many patients and family members ago. Over the years, on more than a few occasions, people have accosted me on the street in

Boston or San Francisco, greeted me like a lost friend in the checkout line of a supermarket in Anchorage or Seattle. They call me by name; they hug me as I make a stab at the right social noises, an effort to buy myself time as I figure out who they are. Sometimes there's an awkward pause while my neurons work overtime, straining for a little sizzle of connection. Sometimes they're kind enough to notice my blankness and offer clues.

But once I place them, it comes back to me in a kind of experiential totality. Who they were, how they were. I feel the heat of the warmers in the intensive-care nursery where I cared for the supermarket lady's six-hundred-grammer, who had a few wisps of bright blond hair. She was sweet but anxious, needed lots of information and assurance. She cried the first time she got to hold the baby, weeks after his birth. It took me twenty minutes to sort out all the lines before and after I slipped the wee bundle into her arms. And her little towheaded preemie didn't make it; it was a brand-new full-term infant she held in her arms next to the frozen foods. The guy I met on First Avenue who asked me with such urgency if I remembered him had missed a curve and hit a tree at high speed, late at night on a deserted country road. I smell the moldy damp of the helicopter's interior, poke a 16-gauge needle into the springy blue rope of a forearm vein, upside down, from my seat in the helicopter. Youth and health had blessed him with huge veins, and his seat belt had kept him from a world of hurt.

I think I see a hitch of recognition as our cardiologist shakes my hand, and I want to ask him if he remembers me, and my mother. But Doreen is launching into report, and our patient is waiting on the table with his coronary artery occlusions, sighing away his fears.

I turn and pass behind glass into the monitoring booth in the corner. It's tiny, with only one chair. I hear him thank Doreen for our good work. He moves off to the table, slips with quick, efficient movements into a sterile gown, mask, and gloves. The staff has prepped the patient, and the cardiologist begins at once to thread a catheter into a groin artery. It's a catheter with a balloon at the tip. Once it is snaked up through our gentleman's trunk, through the secret tunnel of his aorta into his heart, the balloon will be inflated to press the fatty deposits and clotted blood to the wall of the artery, and a stent, an expandable mesh tube, will be placed and left behind to keep the artery open.

Doreen and I shuffle papers and manuals in the booth to carve ourselves a spot to chart. There's quite a bit of information scribbled on overlapping strips of two-inch tape stuck to our blue-suited right thighs. We've got a lot to say.

∽

TUESDAY, JUNE 4, 3:00 P.M.

Yet another rosary from my sisters in my mother's ICU room. Only a day into this odyssey, and how many by now? Ten? I wasn't sure which of the Mysteries they were working their way through on this particular trip around the rosary beads. I remembered Sorrowful and Joyful, but not the rest—I hadn't given them a thought since grammar school, since the last time I owned a little white St. Joseph Missal. Girls' missals were white, boys' were black. The Mysteries were outlined somewhere near the back, under a color drawing of the Virgin in her usual blue-and-white desert outfit. I've said some rosaries in my time, but I always felt the Mysteries were expendable.

But Bernadette and Camille had returned to the Catholic fold, and it was Catholicism on steroids. They observed every arcane particular, and put some of their own idiosyncratic spins on it as well. Over the previous five or six years, as they traversed the choppy waters of their thirties, they had both become immersed in a species of ultraconservative Catholicism that sought to repudiate the reforms of Vatican II. It seemed to me as if they had suddenly acquired a nostalgia for the Middle Ages. The Middle Ages were filled with mud, poverty, social inequities, starvation, and plagues.

Bernadette was once a special-education teacher, Camille a chef. Both sisters are married with children, but they took to wearing dreary clothes that covered them head to foot, along with sandals in winter. Jesus, it seemed, preferred dark and dowdy to colorful and chic. They wore blue cloths on their heads like novice nuns, to signify the religious order of married people they planned to start. Medieval martyrs had become their heroines. They wore large-link chains around their necks to symbolize their servitude to the Lord, hung with many medals, enough to click and clank. They deprived themselves of pleasures, slept on floors. They became capable of using words like *licentiousness* in casual conversation. They opted for homeschooling.

I know my sisters weren't alone. I know there are many, many people who have found a bulwark, in these unsettled times, in religious fundamentalism of every stripe. And my sisters had always been spiritual seekers. We are, in a way, a family of seekers. But I didn't understand all the reasons they'd segued from the open-minded, accomplished, funny women they had been to this cul-de-sac, which to me seemed dark and humorless.

After the first year, I stopped talking to them about it, tried to confine my conversation to topics that didn't ferry us into religious waters. I didn't want the messages from Jesus that Bernadette thought she had for me. I don't believe in the invisible, omnipotent Jesus, but if he should by some chance exist, I'm sure he could speak for himself. So far he hasn't. I couldn't bear the fervent lilt in Camille's voice, the rapt look in her big brown eyes as she warmed to some theme involving purity and virginity. I worried for their mental health. My sisters found

those concerns patronizing and insulting, a reason to feel mar-
tyred.

"Why, this is what Jesus went through when no one would
believe in him," Bernadette told me.

I missed my sisters, who had been best friends. When I tried
to talk with them in the old, familiar ways, they responded with
eagerness to give me spiritual advice and counsel, especially in
the beginning, before I made it plain I wouldn't sit still for that.
And their symbiosis made them stronger in this thing than either would have been alone.

We didn't seem to have a common language anymore.

Even a meal in the hospital cafeteria with them meant enduring a loud, exhibitionist grace, the sort of thing that made
diners in the far corners snap their heads up from their news-
papers. As their voices carried the meal's blessing up to the
ventilation ductwork and out to the hallway, my lips puckered
involuntarily over my cafeteria tray. I felt like I was swallowing
something worse than the hospital meat loaf.

But for years it had distressed my mother that my sisters and
I weren't as close as we once had been. Above all, in her hospital
room, over her potential deathbed, she would have wanted us to
get along. And my mom was Catholic, though a freewheeling,
freethinking sort of Catholic, never the sort of rigid dogmatist
her daughters had become. Still, Mom believed. She believed
especially in the presence and intercession of the Virgin Mary.
I never heard her mention any of the other religious person-
ages—they didn't seem to compute. I think it was her version
of finding something female in the realm of the Almighty. The
Judaic-Christian tradition *is* a little short on feminine power
and presence. But wherever it sprang from, her belief had always seemed to help her. To steady and console her. I knew she
would have welcomed at least *some* of her daughters' rosaries,
and once, to honor that, I would have joined in. Before religion

became a funhouse at a dark carnival; before people I loved went in but didn't seem to come out.

In the most basic ways, my mom had always played fair with me, and I knew she didn't expect me to pray over her at this late date. When I couldn't stand the droning Hail Marys another second, I slipped out for a latte. But I wished I were a smoker. A two-pack-a-day, every-thirty-minutes kind of smoker.

My mother had been dialyzed a number of times, and her weight was way down. That weight was fluid, presumably from her lungs as well as elsewhere, so her kidney specialist thought we could try to get her off the ventilator the following day.

Earlier that day, I had met the cardiologist. Standing in the doorway of Mom's room, he had shared with me a few tidbits of technical information on the various cardiac enzymes and their interpretation. It was a friendly move—aimed, I think, at acknowledging my status as a sort of colleague. But I'm a jack-of-all-trades, not a cardiac specialist, and I forgot the details almost immediately.

"Is the damage extensive?" I asked him. He had done some ultrasound imaging of my mom's heart.

"There's a big section of heart wall that isn't moving," he replied.

I didn't ask him the real question, which was whether we should be doing more, should already have done more. He didn't volunteer any solutions, didn't discuss it in any way. And I still don't know if by not asking, I was acting on or abnegating my conscience. How culpable was I? I didn't want to her die, but I had made a decision the evening she was admitted. I had decided not to put her through it. Not to up the ante, not to push for the full extent of what cardiology might have to offer. In a way, it was letting nature take its course, except that there's nothing natural about the ICU setting to begin with. A ventilator isn't natural. Hemodialysis isn't natural. But if a ventilator will get you through a bad patch, let you live to fight another day, it's worth it. It's what will come after the ventilator that matters.

And I didn't know for sure *what* would come after. Not if we transferred her somewhere for higher-level care, and not if we didn't. If you're looking at permanent brain damage, the hands-off, do-less, withdraw-support decision is easier to make. But that wasn't the case with my mother.

After years in the ICU, you develop a finely tuned sense for the mortal shape of things with your patients, for just how sick they are, how close to death they are. For whether they will, in fact, die of whatever is ailing them. It's a sense that forms, like metamorphic rock, from the inexorable pressures of intellect and experience, and it feels like intuition, but isn't.

It's not infallible. Far from it.

Still, you become a kind of walking algorithm. You take in a thousand pieces of information; you're not even aware of the source of them all. And you come up with a strong impression. The impression comes from the broad strokes—everything you've ever learned or experienced regarding the patient's problems, and how many problems, like dominoes, there are. It also comes from the little details: what the last labs and imaging showed, what the vital signs are doing based on how much fluid and pharmacologic support. It's sensual, based on how patients look, smell, feel to the touch. How their voices sound, if they're able to talk, how much fluid, mucus, or wheezing you hear in their chests. And there's a piece that takes into account some intangibles, like who the patient is, how his life might have led him to the ICU. A seventy-year-old lonely bachelor has different intangibles, different forces acting on him than a thirty-year-old mother of toddlers does.

My mother was much loved. But new worlds, like fractals,

evolve from single decision points, and on Monday night, the night she was admitted, my gut told me no: give her the gift of beginning to let go, even if that gift is the offering of a serpent, an exile from the Garden.

∞

1925

I work at three different suburban bases, but whenever I'm stationed here, at this valley airfield ringed by mountains, I try for a brisk walk between flights, an hour spent prowling around the parked Cessnas and Pipers on the ramp to the runway. I need the exercise, and the only piece of workout equipment we have at this particular base is a broken ski machine. But I also walk because my home is in hills and trees, where vision is truncated, doled out in bits and pieces. The expanse of this place, the light and clarity of it, works on me like a drug.

Even at night. Full dark comes early in November, but we're between rain squalls tonight, and the air on the ramp is crisp and cold. The stars, with their ancient cosmic light, are many. I walk in jeans, jacket, and running shoes; my flight suit, boots, and helmet are laid out and ready on a chair in the hangar. My pager volume is turned up. I'm a little paranoid about missing a page, though Doreen and the pilot striding out in full gear to take their places in the helicopter, which is in front of me on the ramp, might be a clue that a flight is in the offing. I have it timed, how long it would take me to sprint back to the hangar from the apogee of my circuit around the ramp, jump into my flight suit, and zip up my big, black steel-toed boots. Two minutes. I won't delay anybody's transport with that.

My tromp around the ramp is meditative. It lulls some of the edginess I feel at quarters, between flights. Whether I'm awake or asleep, some part of me is always watchful, remains on red alert when I'm on duty, waiting for the high-pitched beep of the pager. So far today, we've had only the one flight. My nerve endings know that more mayhem is out there with our names on it, and I sigh, because it's evening and my body, like everyone else's in the world, is beginning to wind down. I'd rather do my flying in the daytime.

Our cardiologist successfully stented open a couple of branches of our patient's right coronary artery, we learned an hour ago when Doreen called the ICU to inquire about him. He was awake, alert, and doing well. His wife had arrived from their home in the little coastal town and was sitting at his bedside, holding his hand. Doreen and I acknowledged a brief flash of professional satisfaction, along with the hope that he wouldn't re-occlude in the next week or two, as sometimes happens with stents. I dashed off a letter to the sending hospital informing them of the patient's outcome. Another flight closed, another task crossed off the list.

My mother seems close, somehow, as I plod alone around the little planes, all tied down in neat rows. I talk to her, though I don't believe she can hear. I tell her I miss her. I don't tell her I'm not sure I did the right thing for her. It's over and done with, a burden that belongs to me alone. But the stars turn with me, north to south, south to north, and the wind comes up, riffles through my hair, which has been flattened to my scalp by my helmet.

∞

WEDNESDAY, JUNE 5, 12:30 P.M.

Visibility was poor. The marine layer blotted the sun from the sky, shrouded the grounds of the hospital under a damp and monochromatic blanket. Fingers of fog dipped into the tops of the hemlocks. There would be no helicopters flying into that neck of the woods, not unless the fog burned off. I could taste the inlet's salt tang on the air as I caught a few minutes outside after lunch, a respite in the parking lot outside the ER. There were festivities planned for the afternoon—my mom's breathing tube was due to be removed.

I girded my loins, which translated to cradling my latte with both hands, watching county medic units come and go. I amused myself by figuring out which towns they were from. I should have been out in a helicopter, meeting some of those units in the field. I was supposed to work that day, a twenty-four-hour shift, but I'd given the office a heads-up about what was happening with my mom.

Unfortunately, it wasn't a good urban latte—no double shot of aromatic espresso, no creamy head of steamed milk. I would have killed for one of those. Nope, this was the latte of the hinterlands, and I had to make do. The cup was right: thick cardboard, a bright, Italian-inspired design, a sippy lid. But inside, the milk was scalded, the coffee acrid and thin. It tasted like something made in a church basement.

In Mom's room, the tang was of disinfectant mingled with the randomly organic: her sour breath, a whiff from the odd puddle of diarrhea under a patient across the hall. It was dim. There was a wall of window behind the column of ports and electrical outlets at the head of her bed, but the light from it was gray and monotonous. We had to make do with that too.

They had weaned down her ventilator settings and her sedation over the course of two hours, and her blood gases were acceptable. A moment or two to undo straps, and the breathing tube was out.

I held her hand, kissed her forehead. She was warm, and with so much fluid removed by dialysis, a little doughy.

"Hey, Mom," I said. "Here you are."

"Jennifer," she croaked, squeezing my hand.

It was so good to hear her voice, an unexpected relief, fresh water in the outback. I had been holding my breath. I didn't know what to feel, what to hope for. It was one thing to pace the cage of my own thoughts as she lay unmoving in the dimness of her room, a body already lying in state. Another thing entirely for her to open her dark eyes, smile, hang on to my hand for dear life. For a few heady hours, I thought, I *hoped*, that maybe, just maybe, we were going to have her back.

I wish I remembered verbatim what we said that afternoon. There should be a transcript, so I'd have something to hold on to, something tangible. But I have only the odds and ends that float around in memory, flotsam and jetsam.

I remember telling her that all her grandsons had been in to see her.

"Wonderful," she said, her voice raspy. Some of the grandsons were on hand, I think—the older boys, Aaron and Nick, Luke and Jarek. They drifted into and out of her room, and she bantered with them in one-word spurts, letting them do most of the talking.

Bernadette and Camille massaged her feet; endlessly, it seemed. It was something she loved, and needed—her feet hurt from diabetic neuropathy—and I was grateful to them for that. Intermittently they murmured prayers, and I tried not to mind, to push aside the religious animosity I know is a bit irrational on my part.

Mostly I envied the simplicity with which they saw her need and met it. I did take a turn at her feet, but I had to steel myself to do it. Gnarly feet gross me out, plain and simple, and the other dirty little truth is that touchy-feely has been all but bred out of me. Too many people, too many bodies. Massage is too close to the bone. To ask me to rub somebody's feet, even my mother's, is asking for something a little beyond what I have to give.

Mom did okay for a while. Long enough for Berny and Camille to feel they could go home to their younger children for a few hours, and for my father to go with them. He had been a wraith in the corner of the room since the odyssey began, never managing to stay long. He was a poet, a jokester, a backroom philosopher, not often at a loss for words. But for days he'd had little to say.

"It's a lump" was his comment about her situation. He had gestured somewhere between his Adam's apple and his heart. "A lump that doesn't go away."

Of the family, then, I was the only one with her when she started to fail. She began by trying to clear her throat but couldn't seem to do it. I could hear mucus or fluid rattling, and she couldn't cough it out. At first it was intermittent, and she was still able to talk. It sounded like it was in her upper airway. I thought, *Okay, no big deal.* As the minutes ticked by and her attempts to clear it became more constant, her nurse tried to snake a suction tube through her mouth toward the back of her throat.

I kept up a stream of quiet, encouraging nurse-babble to try to get her through it. "I think we can help you out a little bit with this suction tube, Mom. We'll just slip it in along the side of your mouth and get that bit of mucus out. Might make you gag a little, but it'll just take a second."

This sort of patter had been my lot with her for years, through surgeries and colonoscopies and x-rays and doctors' visits. In any medical setting, she was always a hairbreadth away from panicking, an errant word or action away from stampeding right out the door.

Oral suctioning didn't work. It siphoned some saliva and

mucus but didn't make it any easier for her to breathe. Next, her nurse tried going through her nose, a way you can sometimes pass the catheter deeper into the trachea. Much more unpleasant, and I nattered away at fever pitch, my mother's hand death-gripping mine.

The nasal route didn't make things better, either. She sounded wetter and wheezier by the minute. Her heart rate climbed until it was in the 150 range, as it had been the night she was admitted. They switched from a nasal cannula to an oxygen face mask, to give her a higher concentration of oxygen, and gave her albuterol for her wheezing. I began to be afraid she was extending the damage to her heart.

The suction tube, as necessary as it seemed, tipped the scales toward panic for her, as I had been afraid it would. But it was more than panic. Her oxygen saturations were dropping into the 80s despite 100 percent oxygen, and it was becoming clear that she needed to go back on the ventilator.

"Does she *want* to be re-intubated?" her nurse asked me quietly.

The million-dollar question. "I've never been able to get her to say," I told her. "She's blind, wheelchair-dependent, in pain, on dialysis. And her quality of life has been getting worse and worse for a while. Bad things have been happening all spring. But . . ." I shrugged.

The nurse turned to her. "Jo, you're having so much trouble breathing, it looks like we're going to have to put the breathing tube back in," she said. "Is that what you want? Because if you don't want that, we can give you medicine to relax you and take away pain, make you comfortable."

"I don't know," my mother murmured between breaths, the wet knot rumbling in her chest. Her eyes were hooded. "I don't know what that means."

"You've been on the respirator for the past couple of days, Mom. There's a tube that goes into your windpipe to connect you to the ventilator. They're going to have to put it back in."

"I don't remember it," she mumbled. And I'll be damned if I don't think I saw the stony look on her face, the very same one that settled on her during our aborted living-will conversations in my car. The look she got whenever she trumpeted, *Well, when I go, I go. When I kick the bucket, that'll be it for me.*

She was opting out of the discussion.

Maybe I should have been blunt. Maybe I should have said, *Mom, what they want to know is whether you're ready to die.* But I couldn't bring myself to do it. It plain wasn't fair to ask her that question as she struggled for every breath. There are people in this world who *could* make the decision, right there and then, even drowning in their own fluids. People who would never abdicate the right to make that decision. I've met them. But she wasn't one of them.

I put in a quick call to my father from the desk at the nurses' station. "You might want to come back down here," I told him. "She's having trouble breathing again, and it looks like the tube needs to go back in. What do you think?"

He didn't hesitate. "I think we should let her go," he said. "I think she really started to go on Monday, here at home."

The fog had burned off, I noticed, with the phone to my ear. Shafts of sunlight beamed across the nurses' station from the windows of rooms that faced south and west. My mother's room, with a northern exposure, wasn't one of those.

The rays felt warm on my face. Idly, I watched dust motes float inside them.

I thought my dad was right, that she really had started to die on Monday. My professional self was afraid that by putting her back on the ventilator, she might improve just enough to live a broken shadow life for a while. I knew she wouldn't want that. Still, the stony look nagged at me. It told me she didn't seem quite ready to *kick the bucket* either.

"I can relay the message," I told Dad, "but I don't think they're going to take that directive from me. They'll need you to sign, and I don't think they're going to be able to wait until you get here."

"Well." He sighed. "Bernadette and I will be down as quick as we can."

Her room was abuzz with familiar activity. The staff was laying out equipment for intubation. Her kidney specialist had arrived.

"Oh, good, you're here," he said, facing me across her bed. She was no longer up to talking, was in fact beginning to acquire the gray, absent look that comes over people shortly before they quit breathing altogether. "We need to re-intubate."

"Yes, I know," I said. I squared my shoulders, feeling as if I were David taking on Goliath in front of a cast of thousands. "But the question is, should we?"

I felt I had to raise the question. Even though it was my mother, even though I loved her. *Because* I loved her and I didn't want her life to shrink down until it comprised nothing but an unending series of the medical procedures she feared and hated.

He stopped short. "What do you mean?" he demanded.

I hurried through it all again, mindful of her shitty color and the seconds ticking away. "She's in kidney failure, blind, immobile. She has periods of disorientation. She has hallucinations. The sphere of her life has gotten smaller and smaller, and there's less and less good stuff in it. More and more pain. Now she's had a big MI. Our ability to take care of her at home was stretched to the max before this happened. I don't want to save her now just to doom her to life in a nursing home, a life where it takes three strong men to prop her up in a chair for a couple of hours. I know that isn't what she wants."

The respiratory therapist and nurse were following the discussion, turning their heads from me to him, from him to me. They looked like they were watching a ping-pong match.

"Well, she may have to go to a nursing home for a time, but perhaps it wouldn't need to be a permanent condition." He hesitated before launching his next salvo. "And you of all people know that now is not the time to be making these decisions. You should have discussed it with her before now."

I didn't know whether to laugh or cry. I definitely wanted to slap him. "I've tried to discuss it with her. I think you know she is not medically sophisticated, and she wasn't receptive to learning. She wouldn't say what she wanted."

He stared at me again. I didn't know what the deal was. Certainly he had to have faced these questions in his practice before. People with end-stage kidney disease *will* die without dialysis or transplant. There have to be people in this world who make the decision not to embark on dialysis in the first place. There certainly had to be people in his practice who were in my mother's shoes, with problem piling upon problem, the quality of their lives degrading more every month. I wondered why he seemed so uncomfortable with the idea that enough might be enough, that there's a point at which it makes sense to stop intervening.

Maybe he didn't brook much interference from family members with his clinical decisions. And I wasn't trying to interfere, exactly. I didn't know what the right thing was. I don't believe there's an absolute morality in situations like this. We all just do the best we can. I've watched a lot of families grapple with it before me.

(My brother, Kevin, has a different perspective. "I think he just liked Mom," Kevin said, long after it was all over. "She showed up every other day for dialysis in that red coat. And she might have given him a hard time, but she was never boring. She charmed him, in her way. I think he hated to give up on her.")

"Anyway, it's not *your* decision," he was saying at her bedside. "It's up to your dad."

"I just talked to him. He thinks we ought not to re-intubate. He's on his way back down here now."

"Well, I need to have that directly from him," he said. "And," he went on with a particular emphasis, "what about your sisters?" It was clear he hadn't missed the medals and rosaries. "Shouldn't it be a family discussion? I think we need to intubate her now, dialyze her again, and have a family meeting tomorrow after my office hours, talk about what should happen if she doesn't improve."

There was nowhere else for me to go. You can only ring the death knell for your own mother so many times before your courage fails you and people start to wonder what you stand to inherit. I stole a look at Mom's ashen face, shiny with sweat.

"Okay," I said. "That's what we'll do."

But I've never felt more drained than I did at that moment. Not ever. And that is saying something.

I needed a latte. An urban latte with a triple shot. Creamy, hot, and strong enough to zap me back to life. I could smell it.

"I'll step out for a few minutes," I told the troops in her room. "Let you all get on with it." The laryngoscope was laid out on her chest, and I noticed they were opening up an 8.0 tube. Kind of big for someone her size. She was only five-one. Short but mighty, that was my mom. I couldn't help thinking that even with her singer's lungs, I'd have gone for the 7.5.

∞

Bernadette and my father arrived, and Bernadette had brought a priest. In my mother's room, the ventilator hissed and clicked. Her numbers were better. Propofol was back on, and she didn't stir.

My father had just signed a directive not to resuscitate. He and I stood at the desk, planning with Mom's two doctors what should or should not be done if her condition deteriorated further. The cardiologist said she'd had another heart attack.

Bernadette came out of the room. "Father is ready for us now," she said, gesturing toward the priest.

My dad scuttled toward my mom's bedside. I waved Bernadette off. "I need a minute," I told her.

Three years younger but much taller than I am, Bernadette is a woman with physical presence. She had started out in young-adult life as an actress, majoring in drama prior to obtaining her certificate in special ed, and I wish she had continued with acting because she was riveting onstage, outsize. She has beautiful large, hazel eyes that she got from our dad, plentiful wavy hair that's almost the same color as fir bark. She is generous, imaginative. She would give you anything she has if you wanted it. You wouldn't even have to need it, just want it.

My parents had been living with Bernadette for six years, soaking up some of her family's resources, their money, time, and energy. But she'd never once complained or guilt-mongered about it, as she might have. "It works out fine," she'd always said. "They help me out whenever they can. I like having them there."

The flip side to her generosity is that at times, if you don't agree with her, she can come a little unhinged. A key fact to know about her is that she has no problem at all with a scream-fest in public.

She ducked back into Mom's room for about thirty seconds, then approached me again.

"You need to come in *now*," she said with an edge, pointing toward the room. "Father's ready."

I didn't give a shit about Father. And I didn't need her haranguing me to come in and pray. She knew exactly how I felt about that subject.

"I don't want to!" I blurted out before I could stop myself. I'm sure embarrassment flared up my neck and onto my face; I know I thought, *Oh yeah, Jen, that's smooth.* The two doctors exchanged a look.

Normally I would have tried harder. I would have said, *I'll be in as soon as I've finished. You go ahead and get started.* I'd have tried to defuse her, and I'd have reminded myself that in the matter of prayer, it's better to err on the side of generosity than to nurse a grudge like a pugnacious asshole. But even the urban latte I'd found couldn't put me completely to rights after the afternoon's events.

"You don't want to?" Bernadette echoed. Her thick brows beetled together, her mouth thinned. The tone and volume of her voice began to rise. "You don't *want* to?" The unspoken hung between us: *Our mother is dying and you won't even pray for her?*

Yup, that was exactly how things stood. After a lifetime of church choirs and Catholic schools, I could hardly believe it myself.

I shook my head. "I don't want to," I said again. My refusal had metal in it. There wasn't anything I could do about that.

She stared at me. I thought for a moment that things were going to escalate into a real scene. But then she made a noise—*Ptscha!*—and left me at the desk.

I finished talking details with Mom's doctors. *No pressors if her blood pressure falls. No chest compressions.* It was its own sort of tired litany.

When I entered, the priest was standing at the head of Mom's bed, next to the ventilator. His voice was rising and falling in the ordered cadence of prayer. Maybe he was administering the sacrament that used to be called Extreme Unction, which had morphed into the Anointing of the Sick. Either way, it's last rites.

Bernadette and my father stood at the footboard. *Our Father, who art in Heaven, hallowed be thy name.* Their voices, too, reached toward an afterlife, or at least toward some sort of resolution. *Thy kingdom come. Thy will be done, on earth as it is in Heaven.* They each held one of Mom's horny, inert feet. I slipped between them, put my left arm around my father's bony shoulders, my right around Bernadette's waist. *Give us this day our daily bread.* They were warm, and after a moment, Bernadette leaned in toward me. *And forgive us our trespasses, as we forgive those who trespass against us.*

I mouthed the words without sound. *Deliver us from evil.* It was the best I could do.

∞

THURSDAY, JUNE 6, 10:30 A.M.

Exercise had been in short supply all week, and I needed some. It was either that or start drinking martinis before noon. In the softness of that hazy morning, I huffed my way up Day Road on my bike, six miles into the ride, feeling worn and off my game but relieved to be alone. I had to dismount at the entrance to the vineyard for a few pulls at my water bottle. I envy the thoughtless grace of riders who can steer with their knees, clipping along at twenty miles per hour, guzzling water and popping energy bars like they're at their own kitchen tables.

But the vineyard is a natural place to stop, even if you're not a klutz. Heading east on Day Road, you climb to it gradually, emerging from the shade of trees. As you cut out of the steady stream of traffic into the lip of gravel at the entrance, light blasts at you from three corners of the compass—you enter big sky, and something in your cells wells up. Sap, perhaps. Behind the padlocked gate, tidy rows of vines fall away to the south, down a mild slope. There's an empty fruit stand where they sell berries by the flat in the summer—beautiful, ephemeral raspberries that sing on the tongue with cream, ripe with juice that oozes out and stains your palms no matter how gently you handle them. Their season here is so brief you can doze off and miss it.

Once, on a ride with my sons, Gabe and I amused ourselves by naming the spots in our rural-esque neighborhood that we each thought had the most power. Our separate lists dovetailed quite a bit, and the places we take water breaks when we're riding tended to be on them, including the entrance to the vineyard. It mesmerizes me a little, the idea that land itself has power and that some points on the land, perfectly ordinary points, telegraph more power than others.

My children, of course, were divided on the issue. Kieran rolled his eyes at us. His concept of power runs more to the automotive.

"See one tree, you've seen 'em all," he'd said cheerfully, showing nature his back. His eye, as always, was on the rolling iron.

Away to the west, above where Day Road drops back down toward the highway, you can see the Olympics. But clouds obscure the mountains so often in western Washington that when it's clear, they can sneak up on you. *Oh, good,* I thought on that June day, *you guys are still there.* I could see significant snowpack clinging to the slopes. Water for the long, dry summer ahead, hung out into thin air like full saddlebags.

My mother hung out there, too, drugged and ventilated. The hospital's coordinates fixed her in space to the southwest, in the general direction of the Olympics. Close, as the crow flies. Minutes in the helicopter. But because of the peculiarities of topography, because of the nature of islands, inlets, and peninsulas, it was thirty miles by road. I wondered, with a hint of an ache in my gut, how much longer I would be able to place her anywhere.

Like the mountains, she was caught between heaven and earth. *This can't go on, Mom,* I thought.

I was due at the hospital—I had to get going. I finished my water and mounted up for the last third of a mile to the crest of the hill.

As I stood up for the steeper bit right at the top, I was half congratulating myself for how well I was managing overall. I'm used to thinking in an analytical way about life's stressors; it's one of the things nurses do. Hour after hour at bedsides, talking to people, trying to relieve their pain, trying to ameliorate some of their anxieties, meeting their families and friends, you get a feel for what's at work in their lives, and also for what coping abilities they bring to the table. It's a dynamic thing; a manageable challenge one week can be overwhelming the next. Add enough stressors, and anyone will melt down.

Coping depends on a kind of dance, a dance between everything under the sun that taxes a person and the resources that person can summon to deal with it all. By resources I mean extrinsics, like money, shelter, a social network, physical energy. I also mean intrinsics: a sense of humor, knowledge, and optimism. Qualities that are synthesized by neurotransmitters in your brain, shaped through experience, genetics, and luck.

Sometimes you cope through plain stubbornness, which is another name for persistence.

The mortal illness of a parent ranks right up there on the life list of stressors. But I was handling it. There I was, taking care of myself, getting my ride in on a sweet June day. I was still able to luxuriate in the sun on my face. The hill was getting to me—sweat drenched the high-tech fabric of my tank top, and there was that little worm of nausea in the pit of my stomach. But it was only a few more pedal strokes to the top. *This ain't much of a hill,* I told myself. *And you've ridden it about a thousand times. Suck it up.*

The sweat had a mind of its own. It turned cold, never a good thing. I banked right, into a small neighborhood of ranch houses that sit at the crest of the hill. No one was around on a Thursday morning. All was quiet except for the jangle of unseen birds. I managed to stumble off the bike and onto somebody's crabgrass, just in time to retch up all the events of the week, along with a quantity of water that still tasted like vinyl.

"Fuck!" I observed to the empty air. It was strange to understand that pity and guilt, anger and grief were what was glistening on the grass. Strange, but also hilarious, in a dark way. The birds sang on, taking no notice of any of it.

∞

FRIDAY, JUNE 7, 10:00 A.M.

Another two days of dialysis, another umpty-ump pounds of fluid removed from Mom's stubborn, stubby frame. Another try at getting off the ventilator was scheduled for early afternoon.

At ten in the morning I ducked out to the hospital garden. It was a restful spot, a planted terrace with a view of the mountains, and at that moment, it was sunlit and private, the morning air fresh and sweet. I called my father from my cell phone. He was resting at home.

"Dad," I said, "they're gonna take out the tube again early this afternoon. You should probably be here."

We hadn't had the planned family meeting with the nephrologist to discuss the options. We hadn't all been at the hospital at the same time. Christine was flying up from her home in Texas, due in on Saturday night. Bernadette, Camille, Kevin, and I were taking turns at the hospital; we staggered our visits so Mom wouldn't be alone during daytime and evening hours. Our spouses and children milled in and out too. She would have liked that. Above all things, she hated to be alone. I swear she had five children because she was herself an only child and grew up lonely. She wanted to make damn sure her adult life was different.

Even without the family meeting, we seemed to have arrived, without directly discussing it, on more or less the same page about what would happen. If Mom "flew," and managed to stay off the ventilator, we would rejoice and be glad, as the biblical libretto of one of our old choral pieces had it. We'd go to work helping her pick up the pieces. But if she failed again, we wouldn't re-intubate. We'd make her comfortable with sedation and pain medicine and let nature take its course.

"Do you think she's going to make it this time?" my dad was asking.

"No," I said. I hated to be that bald about it, but I was too tired to hedge. My stomach twisted.

"Yeah," he said. "I think it's just her time. I had an argument with Berny about it, but I told her it was my decision."

I nodded, unsurprised. I'd heard about the argument from Kieran, who had been in the room with Bernadette, Camille, and my dad for the fireworks. Kieran thought the religious faction had hammered at him too hard about God's will. "They wouldn't let up," Kieran had told me. "I thought Papa was going to cry. And . . . didn't God decide already? Nana would be dead now if it wasn't for all this stuff attached to her."

"Berny's really close to her," my dad said on the phone. "She's having a hard time."

"Yeah, that's for sure. She imprinted on Mom like a duck." It wasn't the first time I'd had that thought. "They both go on the offense if you don't agree with them." He managed a laugh.

"Maybe she'll surprise us, Dad. You know I don't want to lose her. But if she doesn't . . . I know this is going to sound weird, but I don't want to take away her chance to die a reasonable death. After a while, you ask yourself, are you doing her any favors? If you do manage to save her, what are you saving her for? Things have been spiraling down for her for months now."

He sighed. "I've known her almost sixty years," he said. "And all that time, she was never cruel. She could be a pain in the ear, she'd fuss and fume, but she was generous. Ultimately fair. I could always talk her into being reasonable. But the past five or six months, she's gotten petty. Almost vindictive. No matter what I do, I can't settle her down. I can't make her happy."

There was a small silence. "As far as she's concerned, I've lost all my credibility," he said, trying to make a joke of it.

I knew what he meant, though I think whatever venom she had, she saved for him. She didn't hold back with him. Sixty years of togetherness will do that, I guess. Sixty years of singing and working together, of dating and marrying and arguing and raising children, of burying their own parents and welcoming grandchildren. She made an effort to keep it lighter when she was with me.

I thought they were both exhausted, and that they had many reasons—risk factors, if you will—for depression. But

I also wondered if that isn't how it happens, withdrawal from the world. Maybe your capacity for the good things in life— for laughter, talk, simple satisfaction, for lunch out, for a ride around the countryside, for an electric fight followed by kissing and making up—erodes until there's nothing left but endurance for its own sake.

She failed faster this time. The wheezing and ineffective coughing started within a few minutes, and words were few.

"Make it stop," she said. "Make it stop."

Dad signed another piece of paper. We thanked her doctor for everything he'd done for Mom over the past few years. He left. Nobody fought, about religion or anything else. The nurses started a morphine drip and increased it until she stopped struggling, achieved what seemed like comfortable sleep. We held her hands. My sisters rubbed her feet. I took off her cardiac lead patches and pulled a gastric tube out of her nose. I kissed her forehead, told her I loved her.

While I was gone for a short time in midafternoon, to call Christine in Texas from the parking lot and to get a latte, the rest of the family sang to her. I hope she was able to hear it through the morphine.

Forty years of singing together as a family, and I wasn't there for it. A part of me regrets that. It might have been a form of prayer I could live with. But singing with the family is also a little like massage. Awfully close to the bone.

They moved her upstairs to a private room on a ward in late afternoon, and the staff let us be. We had no way of knowing how long we would need to stand watch and again made plans to stagger our visits so she wouldn't be alone. Camille and I took the first shift, and except for one son for each of us, everyone else went home.

Her oldest, twelve-year-old Luke, stayed behind with us,

along with thirteen-year-old Gabe. Luke and Gabe have been friends since they were babies. They look like brothers, tall and dark, whereas whenever Gabe and blond, stocky Kieran appear together, people tend to ask me if they have different fathers. From their earliest days, Luke's and Gabe's dynamic has been to egg each other on—to climb the eighty-foot tree way back in Luke's woods, then to sidle out near the top onto the skinniest branch that will hold them. To jump off Point White dock into the frigid waters of the sound in January. To tape Roman candles together on the Fourth of July when no adult is watching and light the tangle of fuses.

I'd coached Camille through her labor with Luke, and when she was about four centimeters dilated, I'd gotten a call in her labor suite from Howard, asking me to come home. "Have you lost your mind?" I asked him. He hadn't. Gabe, then thirteen months old, had been standing on a rocking chair facing backward when he bucked it hard enough to tip it over. His fingers were curled over the leading edge of the chair's back when it struck the floor. A tiny digit was lacerated. Fat drops of blood welled up, spattered on the floor whenever Howie eased up on direct pressure.

"Go," Camille had said when she wasn't breathing through contractions. "I'll be fine."

I rushed home, took one look at the gaping edges and the little bit of fat visible in the wound, and knew it needed to be sutured. Howard accompanied Gabe to the ER of a different hospital, one mandated by our HMO, while I returned to Camille, who had *hoo-heed* along without me and was by then seven centimeters dilated. Four hours later, Luke was born, and Gabe was there, asleep on Howard's shoulder, his pretty curls grazing Howard's chin. A pristine white dressing covered the four stitches on his index finger. The following morning, while my back was turned, oblivious to the ER's instructions to keep the wound clean and dry, Gabe dipped his finger in the toilet and swished it around awhile. He seemed to enjoy the feeling of the toilet water as it tickled through the gauze.

In my mother's room now, Camille, spent and pale, sat in a chair by the window, the summer dusk on her face. It took a long, long time for the last dregs of pink-stained solstice light to drain out of the sky. Camille relaxed a bit when Bernadette wasn't around. We hadn't been alone together in ages, and the oldest habits sometimes hold sway. As we talked, her piety receded, and I shelved my truculence about it. Before long, we were making jokes and laughing about stupid things. Gabe and Luke came and went. Halfway through the evening, a hospital security guard brought the boys back to us. His brisk, uniformed entrance brought the real world into the room.

"These boys have been climbing trees out behind the parking lot," he announced. Or were they climbing over the wall, or throwing rocks at stumps? Whatever it was, it was less risky than usual. Worrisome only to hospital attorneys.

Camille and I exchanged glances. *So?* the look said. *They're not smoking crack or breaking windows.* Compared to what was going on in the room, it was pocket change, a little steam blown off. But we both made the appropriate parental noises and sent the guard on his way.

Mom continued to breathe, her mouth a wide *O* of loud deathwatch gasping, punctuated by long pauses. The classic Cheyne-Stokes pattern.

"I've never seen anyone die," Camille said at one point. "I wonder what the moment of death is like." The combined weight of all the Catholic heavenly hosts poised to take our mother seemed to rest on her statement, and I felt myself grow wary. I didn't want to go there. But a long time ago I'd also wondered what the moment of death was like, and had to see.

"I'd like to be here when it happens for Mom. How about you, Jennifer? Do you want to be here?"

"I want *someone* to be here," I told her. "If it's me, that's fine, and if it isn't, I guess I'm okay with that. Mostly, I don't want her to die alone. I don't think anyone should die alone, if you can help it. If I were sure it would only be a few hours, I'd say we should all be here. But it could go on awhile."

"I know you can't predict when it will happen," she said kindly, and I could have kissed her for that.

At 11:00 p.m., hungry, wrung out, and unable to sit there any longer, Gabe, Luke, and I went out for snacks. Camille kept vigil in Mom's room. As we exited the hospital through the ER entrance, I noticed it was a typical Friday night. The waiting room was noonday bright and jammed full. I wondered how soon it would be before we heard the low roar of the helicopter arriving for the first head injury of the evening.

I had promised Camille I'd look for some single-malt scotch, but the state stores were closed. I bumbled around at the nearby Safeway instead, my fatigue suddenly total. Gabe and Luke buzzed up and down the aisles with inexhaustible kid energy, disappearing for minutes at a time, reappearing to chirp out requests. *Can we get this? Can we get that?* They can eat about a million calories a day—the emptier, the better, as far as Gabe's concerned. Luke, I've noticed, has a finer palate, like his mother, chef for some of the best restaurants in San Francisco.

I had been staring at the LSD colors in the potato chip aisle for at least ten minutes, unable to settle on anything, when Gabe skated up to me and stopped short—the cartoon Road Runner teasing Wile E. Coyote.

"Mom, you're dithering," he said. "Make up your mind." Then he vanished again.

Receptors in my brain were crying out for a little sugar shock. We went for the junk—chips and cake, along with root beer and a bottle of cream sherry. Back in the room, we poured our drinks into tiny hospital Dixie cups and toasted Mom with age-appropriate libations. She gasped on, unchanged. She generally didn't drink—half a cup of beer was enough to get her tipsy—but she was a slut for a celebration. She'd have liked our mini Irish wake, complete with grandsons.

Cheap sherry had never tasted so fine. Camille and I smacked our lips and doled ourselves just a touch more. I felt as if we might hang forever in that featureless room on a nameless plane suspended somewhere between life and its alternative. Or maybe the plane has a name. Maybe its name is limbo.

Bernadette arrived at midnight to spell us, as planned. There was a flash of angry disapproval when she saw the bottle. She declined my invitation to have a snort with us, and it hurt to think of the old days when she wouldn't have refused. Mother Superior had returned, and Camille stopped laughing. Without a word said between them, it seemed, Camille had been called on the carpet. I tried not to mind. Hell, I tried not to notice.

In Berny's gravitas, there was grief. I couldn't help but see pain in the set of her jaw and her determination to do things right. What I didn't know but would find out in just a few hours was that that she was pregnant. My bright little nephew Joe was a nine-week tadpole, afloat in primordial soup.

❧

SATURDAY, JUNE 8, 3:00 A.M.

The call came from my father. I'd been home and asleep for an hour and a half.

"Come back to the hospital," he said. "It looks like she's going to go."

I didn't ask for details. I vaulted out of bed, unspeakably groggy. I found clothes and met my husband and sons out by the car. The woods on the verge of the driveway tossed deeper shadows. They moaned and hissed in the breeze.

Howard was holding the phone. "Paul just called," he said. Paul is Bernadette's husband. "Your mother's gone. It was actually about half an hour ago, while Berny was there."

I opened my mouth to say something, but nothing came out. I reached for the men in my life, for Howie, Kieran, and Gabe. They crowded around, shielding me with solidity and muscle. And under a mottled panoply of branches and stars, I cried as though nothing would ever be right again.

∞

0512, KIERAN'S BIRTHDAY

The shrieking pager again. It's a stiletto in my ear, hooking me from the patchy, disturbed sleep I fell into a couple of hours ago.

"Good morning, Four." Tom's voice from dispatch is tinny. Sound quality on these pagers is about as good as it was on those tiny old transistor radios people took to the beach in the 1960s. "Forty-year-old male, MVA."

I thumb the button, and it kills the static that follows his message. This will be our fourth flight since 0900 yesterday. A busy shift. And we're going out to the little hospital on the coast again, this time for a patient with injuries from a motor vehicle accident.

Trying to ignore the nausea of sleep deprivation, I pull on my flight suit and wrinkle my nose. After three flights, it's hygienically challenged, as am I. But they weren't bloody flights, and nobody vomited on me, so I deem it clean enough. It's too late to transfer all the equipment in my pockets to a fresh one anyway. I can hear the telltale whine—the night-shift pilot, Brad, has the rotors cranking already.

We're all exhausted, and nobody talks as the aircraft lifts into the cool and rainy darkness. Doreen and I already know it's my turn to take report on this patient. I hope he's not too broken, for both his sake and ours. From the little we've heard, he could be anywhere on a long continuum. He could be bleeding out from aortic trauma, or he could have a fractured femur. We'll sort it out when we get there.

The fallow stillness of predawn presses down on the land. It won't last long. The cornfields surrounding the airport are a black void below us, but they're limned by the orange sodium lights and neon of the Safeway plaza, and there's an increasing stream of headlights on the freeway heading south toward the city. The first worker bees are headed toward the hive.

Out on the Puget Sound, the world is a milky, murky blur of cloud and water, framed by the steel and windows of the aircraft. Doreen and I shiver and shift in our seats, trying to find positions of comfort. We ball ourselves into our coats to stay warm. Sleep keeps trying to seduce me again, steal its way back behind my eyes with wanton dream images that slide into the stream of my waking thoughts. *I haven't shopped for Kieran's gifts, and we flew our asses off. I can't believe he's seventeen. Maybe I can go to the bike shop later, after a nap. That dark shadow to my left must be Marrowstone Island. Lots of boats twinkling down there on the water this morning.*

Goddamn it, Oakland just scored again. I've slipped into the warm bath of an Indian summer day. I'm in the left-field grandstand at Boston's Fenway Park. The neon Citgo sign, a major landmark of my childhood, rises like a beacon beyond left center field.

But then a small plane flashes in the void just half a mile away, too close for comfort, and I start fully awake. I haven't been watching for aircraft or listening to radio transmissions—both are part of my job. Three pairs of eyes and ears are better than one when it comes to avoiding midair collisions.

"Traffic at ten o'clock, level," I say into my mike, though Brad would have to be blind to miss it.

"Got it, thanks," Brad replies, deadpan.

More sodium lights ring the paper mill. Its plume of steam glows orange, and after a minute, Brad circles to land on the rooftop pad. It's an apron of concrete with a walkway to the enclosure for the elevator, which is brightly lit at this hour. I can see our welcoming committee, a building engineer with a gurney, waiting just inside the door.

While Brad begins to power down the engines—shutting them down abruptly reduces engine life—I twist the steel ring that pops my door open. A clean, cold wind sweeps in, and it feels sweet on my face. I hop out, grab the small D cylinder oxygen tank that during flight is secured to a bulkhead next to the door, and strap it down tight on our stretcher. The nose of the helicopter, as Brad has positioned it, points east, and I can see the rain we flew through, huge masses of clouds passing away toward the Cascades, toward first light.

Keeping close to the body of the aircraft to avoid the rotor tips, shaking my shoulders to stay loose, I do a kind of pimp swagger through the sonic gelatin of vibration and thunder, around the front of the helicopter toward the right side. Toward Doreen, who is strobe-lit as she offloads the defibrillator and begins to pull out the stretcher.

Fifty feet down and a mile to the west of where I'm standing, a Catholic cemetery dreams in darkness. A white marble Virgin presides over it under the trees, I know. It's a cemetery affiliated with the church my mother once attended. The last church she sang in. If there were any justice in this life, still-potent echoes of her voice would be floating around its rafters—the one thing she regretted about singing was its transience. Nobody lines up with the latest technology to record church musicians. And recording, she believed, changed the sound. It was less than the highest expression of the art.

"If you paint a landscape or embroider a pillow, you can put it in your parlor and keep it forever," she used to say. "But with singing, you work for years to stand up and sing a note, a *great* note, and then, poof, it's gone."

In the great neuronal divide between my work and my life, in this present-tense, roaring, rooftop kaleidoscope, I've forgotten until this very second that I've come to her town. The only spot on the map where I can now place her, her final repository.

I don't know where her soul is, or her voice. But her DNA is here.

I grab my side of the stretcher and together, our faces winking on and off in phase with the lights on the tail rotor, Doreen and I slide it out and onto the engineer's gurney. There's no time to wax poetic about a beloved son who's growing up, or a mother I've just begun to miss, a final shape of grief I'll be tracing for the rest of my life. Some fellow traveler, with his unknown traumas, is waiting. I can't linger.

Chapter Ten

Theories of the Universe

Our dad's dentures went to the dump. They'd been ill-fitting for years. I think he might have had them since the army, which would date them from the Korean conflict. But he had lost so much weight they wouldn't go into his mouth when they laid him in the casket. Or did we—my sisters and brother and I—decide at the moment of parting, after he was loaded into the funeral home's van, that he'd be more comfortable in perpetuity without them? Did we discuss whether he'd want to chew in the afterlife? I can't quite remember. We might have. It's certainly not beyond us.

I did think—I worried a little—that my sister Camille would want to keep them as a memento. Or that I would be asked if I wanted them. But after he died, when we were cleaning his room—her basement family room—she picked them up in their blue plastic case. I saw her lips twist, a moue that was mirrored on my face whenever I had to handle the things. And she didn't even say anything. They just sailed into the maw of the big black garbage bag sitting squat in the middle of the floor.

The bag already held some of the detritus that accrues around death at home. Blue-backed waterproof pads, adult-sized diapers. Zinc-based butt cream with lidocaine, a local anesthetic, to numb the pain from the bedsore. A Foley catheter, skuzzy at the tip, and the stained bag the urine drains into.

Things you won't need again unless somebody else is dying in your basement. Things you need to clear away to move on.

They were things I associated with my work. I'd wanted to care for my dad in his last days, and I did, though Camille and her family assumed the biggest share of the burden. But a dissenting, recalcitrant, poltergeist part of me was aghast at the blurring of the border between work and home.

∞

Pacifica, California, 1989. Probably twenty hospitals within a twenty-mile radius. I worked at one of the biggest ones. Who knows how many urgent-care centers and doctors' offices? Urologists were certainly thick on the ground.

My father was having trouble with his prostate. He couldn't pee. He wanted to know what I thought.

"See a urologist, Dad," I said. "If you want, I'll ask around and get some names for you today."

He balked, as I'd expected him to. "I don't want to see any doctors. It's all pills, pills, pills or cut, cut, cut with doctors."

These were the first few bars of a long, familiar riff. Howard and I used to have a joke about how easy it was to push the buttons of some our family members: *Call 1-800-Dial-a-Diatribe! Press 1 for the Health-Care System diatribe. Press 2 for the You're Late with My Birthday Present, Ergo You Have No Love or Respect for Me! diatribe. Press 3 for Real Musicians Aren't Appreciated in This Country.*

The health-care rant was my father's, and it was about how doctors and the health-care system are mechanized, depersonalized, fragmented, greedy, brutal, and in thrall to pharmaceutical and medical supply companies. It was about how there is no innate respect within the health-care community for the body's ability to heal itself, and no allowance for nature to take its course.

I don't disagree with all of it. There are times and places

when each of those charges is true. It *is* a system, and systems have limitations, and so do the people in the system. There are economic forces at work, and sometimes greed. But my dad's complaints aren't uniformly and exclusively true. And this was occasionally difficult over lunch with him, given what I do. Given that I am a part—an agent—of the health-care system. He liked to goad me about it.

I would counter that there's a point at which people can't heal themselves. Most people turn to mainstream medicine when they are ill or injured, I'd say, and somebody should be there when they do. *Okay, Dad,* I'd said once, *you're me. You are in the delivery room, and out pops a baby who is fifteen weeks early and weighs five hundred grams. If nature takes its course, the baby will almost certainly die, and that might be for the best, because if we intervene, she might later bleed into her brain or have other problems that will plague her and her family throughout her life.*

Yet she is lying on the warmer table, tiny and whole and beautiful in her way, and she is breathing on her own. She's a little gelatinous, also a little fierce. She's fighting to cry: a breathy, mewling cry. She starts off a ruddy red, nourished with bright oxygenated blood through the umbilical cord. But you have to cut the cord, and as her breathing becomes labored and falls behind her metabolic needs, she'll begin to turn blue. If you're me, Dad, do you watch her struggle? Or do you dive in, try to apply what you know to help her?

On balance, Dad, I say you apply what you know. Even if it involves tubes and lines and pain for the baby, even if you can't predict the outcome. I'd expected him to at least concede that I had a valid point. We were in his car, which was something like a 1978 Datsun B210, continuing a discussion that had begun over lunch. My father preferred greasy spoons named after people, hole-in-the-wall restaurants like Margie's, Bill's Place, Nancy's. We were driving down the Great Highway past the San Francisco Zoo on a typical day in the fog belt, the surf shushing from

Ocean Beach to our right. I snuck a sideways look at him. His white hair stuck out from under a golf cap (though he never played golf); I could see the set of his chin under his long white beard. To my surprise, he was *pissed.*

Well, you've just negated everything I've ever stood for, he thundered at the wheel. In spite of all my previous exposure to the diatribe, it felt like a non sequitur. I didn't understand how my choice to intervene in the delivery room negated *him.*

Except that I was a daddy's girl until I grew up and out, except that he had a streak of the wizard and the alchemist in him, a talent for articulating all sorts of difficult, subtle things, and I understood that. Loved that about him. Except that for many years, I was a sounding board for all his offbeat theories of the universe.

Except that he did have a talent for healing himself. He had never seen a doctor in living memory. He was spry and wiry. He rode a bike to work in the early 1970s when it was an anomaly for anybody past childhood to be seen on a bike. He practiced yoga daily. He could do both a headstand and a handstand when he was fifty. Left to his own devices, which is to say, away from my mother, his diet devolved to pumpernickel bread and peanut butter, or raisin bran.

After his mother died in 1981 of a sudden stroke, just two weeks after he'd moved away from her, moved all the way from Boston to San Francisco, he had an attack of what looked like some form of arthritis. Every joint was stiff and sore. He was hardly able to move and he wouldn't take so much as an aspirin. I'd offered an entrée to the health-care system then too, and he'd turned me down.

It's just grief, he said. *I'll get over it if you give me some time.* And over time—a lot of time, many months—he did get over it.

Did he heal himself, or was it stoicism carried to the nth

degree? In his living room in Pacifica, 1989, after I offered the names of urologists, after he barked that he didn't want to see a doctor, he turned to my brother, Kevin, who was twenty-four at the time. Kevin was living in Berkeley but was nevertheless the family mechanic, second class. To Kevin fell the role of helping my father patch together a never-ending series of Datsun B210s. One of them had no key or ignition as we know it; you had to hot-wire it to start up in the Safeway parking lot. We all thought that was great fun.

"How about if we take a little ride down to the auto-parts store, Kev, see if there's some sort of tube I can stick up there, drain myself out. There has to be something there that'll work."

I knew he was at least half serious, and on my side a tiny mental movie—a cautionary health film—played out in microseconds: large-bore automotive plastics coated with toxins, sliding against tender internal flesh. Pus, edema, millions of swarming cartoon bacteria. But the phrase "lube job" also leaped to mind, and I burst out laughing. So did Kevin.

"Uh, I don't think so, Dad," Kevin said.

∾

I was drowsing in the semi-dark, upstairs in my little Jenny Lind bed, tucked into the corner of my bedroom in our house in Massachusetts, on Revere Beach, a bedroom that would be remodeled into the kitchen section of an open kitchen/living room in just a year or two. My father was rubbing my back and singing:

> *Sleep my child and peace attend thee*
> *All through the night.*

It was a beautiful, rich, high tenor—it flowed like balm over the bed. I felt safe, utterly safe, and loved. He rubbed my back all through the song, dipping down over my buttocks, which felt good at first, really good, until I remembered that the bum was a verboten area, off-limits. Then it didn't feel so good.

I was a three-year-old just out of the zip-up pajamas with rubber feet, and I didn't know how to tell him that. And if I had told him, he would have scoffed.

∞

Then I was four and we had just gone to United on the Lynn-way, our family grocery store. I was in the backseat of our 1963 Rambler convertible, the only new car we would ever own. There was a black-haired baby in a plastic carrier in the front seat, no seat belt, of course. The baby was probably Christine. As we looped down past the Point of Pines fire station, less than a mile from home, I passed what I thought was a fart, but to my dismay, it came out solid. I hauled myself up to a standing position on the transmission hump between the seats. I didn't want it to squish between my butt cheeks.

"Sit down," my father hissed.

"I can't," I said.

"Why not?"

"There's poop in my pants, Daddy. I thought it was bubbles," I added, not knowing the correct terminology, "but it was poop."

I wasn't sure he would understand what I meant by bubbles. I didn't know if the same thing had ever happened to him. I was just beginning to sort out body functions.

"Do you know about bubbles, Daddy?" I asked, leaning over the front seat. My lower lip stuck out of its own accord, and I started to cry. It seemed like such an awful thing to do, to poop in my pants when I was as old as four. And crying made it worse, much worse.

"Oh, yes," he said immediately. His voice had shape-shifted from irritated to amused to kind. "Don't worry about a thing. You don't have to cry! We'll be home in just a minute."

Once we were home, he cleaned me up in what seemed like nanoseconds, deft, sure, and circumspect. Almost half a century later, I still feel grateful.

∞

The July day was torpid, filled with the smells of grass, sea breeze, coconut oil, and salt, the essences of summer. We were hosting the annual picnic for the adults' and children's choirs—about sixty people—from Notre Dame de Pitie in Cambridge, where my parents were the organist and choir director. My mother stayed home with Bernadette and Christine, who were still babies, and entertained the most sedentary choir members. Some of the others opted for the beach across the street.

Some wanted to go to the amusement park, two miles south of our house, down Revere Beach Boulevard. It wasn't one park, actually. It was a series of individual rides and mini-midways scattered along the beachfront, with a history dating back to the nineteenth century: Hurley's, the Hippodrome, the Mickey Mouse, the Haunted House. We didn't go there very often, despite its proximity—we didn't have a lot of money for extras like amusement parks. But I twirled around, completely stoked, when Dad asked me if I wanted to go with him. I *loved* the rides.

The choir members scattered on the waterfront, and Dad and I centered on Hurley's, a small park with about ten rides. First I rode the baby boats. These were dories with loads of preschoolers floating around and around a six-foot-wide circular canal. The other kids spun the wheels on the boats and made a ruckus ringing the bells, but I knew it was fake. I knew I could reef on the wheel all day long and it wouldn't change the course of the ride one iota. I could walk faster than those boats piddled around the tank.

I was eyeing a ride that had three cars at the bottom of each of four vertical stalks, an adult ride that whizzed into corners and changed direction at high speed, when Dad asked, "So, do you want to go on the Cyclone?" Clearly he had noticed I was bored with the boats.

I had no idea what the Cyclone was. I was four years old, on the cusp of reading, but I didn't read reliably yet. At that moment, I felt the lack in my bones. The whole world was encoded with neon signs and lines of text; the meaning of *everything* lay in reading. I made a promise to myself to memorize the names of the rides at Hurley's before the end of the day, but in the meantime I said yes to the Cyclone. I was sure it was the whizzing ride.

But Dad took my hand and led me in another direction. It wasn't until we were walking up the stairs and along the ramp, under spooky old boards with cracks of bright light between them, walking right under the thunder as the cars hit the nadir of a hill, that I realized what I had gotten myself into.

It was the ancient, white-skeletal, mile-high backbone of the beach, the mother of all rides. It made teenage boys—man-boys with perpetual sneers and perpetual cigarettes hanging from their lips, boys whose entire lives were devoted to looking tough—scream as if they were dying.

There was white noise in my mind, shock that my dad would actually suggest the roller coaster. My imagination failed when I thought of climbing hundreds of feet to the top of the hill in a tiny, open car. I couldn't see myself rounding that apex, or imagine what might happen on the other side of it.

But I wasn't about to back out. And Dad didn't look scared. I took my cue from him, squared my shoulders.

"Are you with me, sweetheart?" he said suddenly. A native Bostonian, he dropped the *r* in *heart—sweethaht*—and his use of endearments was always a little ironic.

"We don't have to ride it, you know. We can do it another time." He didn't say *when you're older*, but I heard it.

"Do *you* think I'm big enough, Daddy?"

For a second he looked as though he'd like to take me back to the baby boats, but then he laughed.

"Yes, I do, dear heart," he joked instead. "You'll be fine."

We sidled into the car. A gruff man with untidy gray hair and brown teeth snugged the metal bar down across the top of our legs. It fit tight across Dad, but there was a sizable gap between my thighs and the bar, and my feet stuck out straight, years and many inches of height away from reaching the floor. The brown vinyl seat was hot and sticky.

The man worked his way up the rest of the chain of cars, then signaled to another man standing behind a dais at the front of the platform. With a creak and a jerk, we were under way.

Dad put his left arm around me. I grabbed hold of the bar, a death grip. We dropped down into a black, weathered tunnel, cold as a freezer in spite of the day's heat. I had a second to notice the dank smell of mold and earth and got a whiff of something that made me think of the Boston trains and old pier pilings. Creosote. Then, with a huge ratcheting sound that seemed to penetrate bone marrow, we burst into sunlight and onto the great hill.

My heart skipped several beats; I felt cold and clammy, out of body. I had no idea what death meant—so far in my life only ancient Uncle Salvy had died, and after a while my mind had stopped worrying at the problem of where he had gone. But from somewhere deep in my brain's primitive limbic system I wondered if I was going to survive the roller coaster. Surviving felt counterintuitive. Yet my father's arm was around me, a constant. An absolute.

And then I had a sort of brain wave, from a center somewhat higher than the limbic system, a center that trumped the limbic system, and though I couldn't know it then, it has served me often throughout my life, whenever I've been the least bit scared. As the car chugged up the hill, I realized that I was, in fact, alive—not just alive but fine—and I understood, though I didn't have the words for it, that panic didn't have to rule the day. I saw I could make a choice about the cold fist in my gut and the roaring in my ears. I could ignore them, for one thing.

I relaxed just enough to feel the sun on my arms, warm after the tunnel. There was a brief interlude, a few seconds, probably—enough—to savor the lightness of the air as we climbed right toward the sky.

It was the first time I'd been more than a few feet off the ground in my life. I could see all the way out to sea, I could see the entire three-mile sweep of gray sand beach, I could see the terminus of the northern subway line, a toy Wonderland train station with its tiny parked cars way down below us.

This is what a bird knows, I thought, and then I wasn't at all panicked anymore. Then I was exhilarated. A primal exhilaration. It felt old, as old as the mysterious earth I'd smelled under the roller coaster.

I snuck a glance at Dad's clean-shaven face. His hair, prematurely gray, was flapping in the breeze, and I saw that he was grinning. He had clearly left behind his daily constraints; he looked *wild*.

"Get ready to scream, honey child," he whooped in my ear as we rounded the top of the hill, a hundred feet of sheer drop in front of us. "Screaming is practically required."

Then the bottom fell out of the world, and screaming took care of itself.

———

As we walked away from the Cyclone, toward car and home, baby sisters and choir members, hamburgers and hot dogs, we passed the whizzing ride.

"Daddy," I asked, pointing, "what's that called?"

"The Scrambler," he said. "We can ride it next time.

∞

My father drove me to school many mornings—St. Mary's High School, Lynn, Massachusetts. After third grade at Our Lady of Assumption in Chelsea, where I had been going to school the day Kevin was born, my parents had taken new positions as music directors for a large parish in Southbridge, a town in south-central Massachusetts. We had lived there for five years. In the middle of my freshman year of high school, we'd returned to the house on Revere Beach.

School started at 7:50 a.m., early for me, but Dad was a morning person, and on the way to school he liked to expound on things while I was pinned in the passenger seat like an insect on an exhibit board. One of his theories of the universe—a theory he liked to twit me with—was an unusual variation of "shit flows downhill." He called it the angel-defecation theory.

"Our shit fertilizes the earth," he would announce. "The angels' shit is what fertilizes us." He could pontificate in this vein for quite some time, about how rich the earth is because we and other beings defecate on it, how it makes everything grow, and all life—all creation—flows from it. And what the angels excrete, in his theory, stimulates all our best thinking, our art, our music, our poetry. What the angels excrete is not organic—it's ethereal, etheric. It's energy.

"Oh, for God's sake," I used to say. "Have some pity." I hadn't discovered morning coffee yet and it was always way too early for angels and defecation. I don't think he believed in angels, in actuality—at least not in any traditional way. But he was on a roll most mornings, trying to get a rise out of me, and talk of ether and spirit, of cherubim and seraphim, shit and piss battered my eardrums all the way to the front door of my school. I pretended to be bored.

∞

How much of me comes from Dad? How many of my synapses are imprinted from his? My father and I did two things together for most of my life. One of them stemmed from the fact that we both loved the piano, but (in contrast to my mother) neither of us played very well. We sucked, as a matter of fact. My father was better than I was, but he had taught himself to play as a teenager—no money for lessons. I took eight years of lessons but had never practiced enough to sight-read accurately. Our solution: we both sat down at the piano, and we each played one hand. My mother often sniffed that we both had talent, and it was a shame we were too lazy to improve. But she also sometimes said, "Well, he taught himself. Pretty good for no training."

We played Bach, mostly. I still have our tattered old copy of *Bach for Keyboard:* the French Suites, the English Suites, the Goldberg Variations, Two-Part Inventions, and Three-Part Sinfonias. Sometimes I'd play right hand, sometimes left. Sometimes we'd play the same piece twice, switching hands. With Bach—and with only one hand to worry about—I could feel the spark and the sparkle in my brain and my fingertips. It mainlined itself in my bloodstream: the syncopation, the changes, the voices, the playful variations, the ornamentation, the speed. Both Bach and my father could manage merry, brainy, and sad, all at the same time.

The other thing we did was the *New York Times* crossword puzzle. We preferred the crosswords from Eugene T. Maleska's reign as puzzle editor to those from Will Shortz's, but my dad, an inveterate newspaper buyer, would save a crumpled Saturday, the week's hardest, for whenever we got together. Huddled on sofas in Massachusetts, New York, California, and Washington, in all his old cars and mine, in the seats of waiting rooms, on ferries, and in choir lofts during endless, windy sermons, we'd argue over who got to write the answers, in black fountain pen and, later, in thick roller-ball ink. I could supply the answers to newer, trendier clues. He had an elephantine memory for literary and classical references, plus lifestyle clues from the era before I was born. Our brains, reaching into inner space to make an arcane language connection and drag it out into the light of a dull weekday, worked alike.

∞

Every so often, my father would ask me if I could get him a urinary catheter from the hospital, and in this way I would know that he was still having problems with his prostate. In 1989, once Kevin nixed the plan for the auto-parts store, Dad did go to an urgent-care center, which was a start but not a substitute for ongoing care. The care he received from a urologist would not have been perfect. It would not have considered every bump and knot in his psyche, or every kink in his genome. It would have been neither as personal nor as disinterested as he wanted it to be. But a urologist, had my dad given him the chance, could have seen to it that my father's bladder emptied itself on a regular basis.

In the end, I suspect Dad ignored the medical advice he was given at the urgent-care center. Somehow his treatment boiled down to saw palmetto, a plant that has been shown to improve prostate symptoms, but in his case—if he even took it—it didn't help. For him, it was magical thinking for prostates.

∞

After my mother died, my father slept much of the time. My mother, with her end-stage kidney disease and two years of hemodialysis, had always been cold. Suddenly, after seventy-five years of thin jackets and the cold breeze in his face, my father was too. He barked at me to shut the window in the car, something he had never done before in his entire life. He seemed to be taking on my mother's peccadilloes, and I wondered if this was some strange grief reaction. But he had also been losing weight for a long time, and once she was gone, his weight loss accelerated. He was in and out of the bathroom every five minutes and looked miserable. He hinted that it was his bowels as well as his bladder, which if true was a new wrinkle to the story. I didn't know what to do for him.

My mother died in June. In September, my dad planned a trip east to see his sister Chickie, nearly eighty years old and living in New Hampshire. A few days before he left, I went shopping with him to buy him some clothes that fit. We had lunch at Elsie's. He ate a few bites of it. He looked anemic—extremely pale, with dark patches under his eyes and a sick green cast to his skin. He was out of breath at the pace of a leisurely stroll, stopping to rest every ten or fifteen feet, whereas six months before I had seen him vault over a turnstile.

A few days before our shopping trip, I had talked to my own family practitioner about him. I'd explained a little about my father's worsening problems and his long-standing antipathy toward the health-care system.

"I know he's had prostate symptoms for at least thirteen years," I had said to David. "And now it sounds like he's having some bloody diarrhea."

I had asked him if he'd accept my dad as a patient, assuming I could get Dad to agree.

"I'll be happy to see him, but I can tell you right now, I'll have to refer him on," David had said.

This I knew, but I still thought it would work best if Dad could have a point of entry with someone who knew a little of the story.

"And," David had added, "that first year after the loss of a spouse is tough. A significant number of people who have been married a long time die in the first twelve months after the death of their spouse."

This I did not know. But maybe I was beginning to intuit it. One large study fixed the percentage of men who die within eighteen months after the deaths of their wives at 13 percent. If you're elderly and the primary caregiver for a disabled spouse, these factors also increase your risk of dying.

At lunch, I put it to him as bluntly as I could.

"Dad, I understand you don't want to be fucked with. But you look bad to me. If you have something that will kill you no matter what anybody does—some nasty cancer, something that requires a lot of invasive treatment for an uncertain outcome—I understand if you don't want to go down that road."

He nodded, listening.

"But I think it'd be an awful shame for you to die of something that is easily treated. You could live ten good years or more. You could do some of the things Mom wasn't able to do and didn't want to do. You're not like her. You've never had diabetes, never had high blood pressure, you've never been overweight. Your heart seems to be good. You could be a spry eighty-five-year-old.

"You could learn to sail. You could hike in the mountains," I went on. I heard the entreaty in my voice.

"Do you really think so?" he said. "I'd like to hike."

"I'll hike with you," I said. "Here's my thought, Dad. You can see a doctor, and you can say yes to some things and no to others. It doesn't have to be all or nothing. I'll help you negotiate it if you want me to. But at least find out what's wrong."

I told him I'd talked to David about him and that I'd make an appointment if he agreed.

"After I see Chickie," Dad said, finally. "I'll do it when I come back from New Hampshire."

I didn't see how he could fly to New Hampshire in the state he was in. But I didn't see how I could obstruct it either. It was clear he was dead set on going. We were alike that way, Dad and me—stubborn and resourceful about what we want to do, unwilling to let anybody else dictate what is and isn't possible, able to put up with a fair amount of hardship, perhaps more hardship than many people would consider reasonable. I learned from him how much you can do—just how far you can take any endeavor—if you're willing to accept some inconvenience, imperfection, uncertainty, and pain. If you're willing to roll the dice.

The plane trip over and back was a "little tough" because he couldn't get to the bathroom easily, Dad said. But he felt it was worth it to see Chickie. I didn't speak to her myself, but I heard from her daughter, my cousin Kathy, that she had been appalled at how sick he'd seemed to be and shocked that we had allowed him to travel alone.

I suppose one of us could have gone with him. But what could we have done for him?

And I knew he didn't want us along. He didn't want some well-meaning blunderbuss of a daughter at the table, changing the character of the talk over the Lipton tea and doughnuts.

At the end of September, he kept his word and saw David, who somehow managed just the right blend of concern and respect for Dad's limits. The stat labs at the clinic showed that he had a hematocrit of 25, anemic, along with evidence of kidney failure: a serum creatinine of 12, sky-high, and a high potassium, which is dangerous because it can precipitate a lethal heart rhythm. He was making urine but not clearing waste products very well.

He was admitted to the hospital. In the ER, they did an ultrasound of his bladder and kidneys, which to my untutored eye showed urine backed up into both kidneys from a bladder swollen bigger than my head. They inserted a Foley catheter into his bladder and out gushed a liter and a half of urine, despite the fact that he had urinated just prior to the procedure.

I wondered how long—for how many years—he had been walking around with a bladder bigger than my head. *Since 1989,* whispered the imp in my limbic system.

Kieran and I took Dad to the urology clinic on Veterans Day, where he had a finger stuck in his rectum one too many times. Thereafter, he refused to return—for a prostate biopsy or anything else.

By this time, he had a stock of clean in-and-out catheters with which to drain his bladder several times a day. He still slept a lot; he still looked pale, he was still thin. But he went out for coffee; he snuck into my house when none of us were home and left baked goods in my kitchen. He played the trumpet, he played the piano, he went to bookstores. I hoped for time, and some form of recovery.

After my mother died, Dad continued living in the studio apartment Bernadette had created from her family room, but in mid-November, right around the time my dad swore off urologists, my nephew Joseph—the newest member of the extended family, the one whose existence we'd learned about the same night Mom died—was born. This made six children for Bernadette and Paul in a small three-bedroom house. One day in December, Dad came to visit, bearing his familiar pink bakery box of doughnuts. He placed it in the center of my kitchen island, like an offering. He perched himself on the edge of the sofa in my small family room.

"I think Berny and Paul need that room downstairs," he said. "The kids are getting bigger. I think I should find someplace else to live." He looked aslant at me, out of the corner of his eye, obliquely beseeching.

Uh-oh, I thought. I knew he was really asking if he could live with me. My house is 2,200 square feet, for four of us.

In the ether around me, I felt the specter of generations of Boston-area ancestors, Catholic immigrants from Ireland and Italy. People with many children and little money whose mode of survival was to band together to live in extended family tribes: grandparents, uncles and aunts, sisters and brothers, sisters-in-law and brothers-in-law, first cousins, second cousins, and sometimes the odd family friend. They—we—lived in South Boston, Charlestown, the North End, Everett, and Revere. Until I left, first for college in upstate New York, and finally, in 1980, when I was twenty-two, for San Francisco, I lived with my parents and siblings, yes, but also my maternal grandparents and my great-uncle.

It was a rich, generous way to grow up. It made sure no one starved, no one was ever homeless, no one was alone.

And I hadn't been alone in San Francisco for long. The next sisters down the line from me, nineteen-year-old Bernadette and eighteen-year-old Christine, were at loose ends, ready for some new phase of their lives to start. Bernadette had attended college for a year as a drama major but had had a dustup with the head of the department and decided to leave. Christine, who had always been a hellraiser within the educational system, was just out of high school, working as a bookkeeper.

I invited the two of them to move out to San Francisco to live with me. I thought of them as friends; we had already been roommates. They came. Bernadette found a job at an upscale shoe store, a job we laughed about, since she of all people cared very little for fashion or shoes. Christine became a teller at a downtown bank. We moved in to a rundown, six-room flat in a haunted old Victorian on Turk Street, at the western edge of the Western Addition.

Within six months, our parents decided to join us.

I was secretly appalled. Living with two of my sisters was one thing. We were equals, more or less. I had moved to San Francisco for independence—the whole point was to live on my own as an adult. I did not want to live with the entire family tribe until I married or died. The very idea conjured the image of maiden great-aunts on both sides of the family, women who lived out their lives and died in the same house under the iron fists of their parents. It was exactly what I had moved west to avoid.

Yet I didn't know how to say no to my own parents. I didn't even know how to insinuate no. To say no would have meant, in family terms, that I was a self-serving, hedonistic bitch who wouldn't give back now that she was an adult. *A product of your times*, my mother used to say whenever we disagreed on contemporary music, or sex, or on any of the many other icebergs floating in the generation gap back then. *We're just shit you want to scrape off your shoes*, my father would say whenever I left home, plying guilt as if it were the mortar between bricks.

So in November of 1980, Camille and Kevin flew out to live with us on Turk Street. I signed them in to George Washington High School, in the outer Richmond District. And in February of 1981, my parents packed up, left my grandfather and blind

Great-Uncle Franky in the downstairs flat on the beach, and drove a moving truck three thousand miles across the country to San Francisco.

It's not what most parents would do. And the motives of parents are one of the enduring mysteries of existence for the children who follow. But I *think* my parents had had enough of hardship, enough caring for their own parents, who had been ill and needy for nearly a decade by February of 1981. They had never had the resources or leisure to travel—some of the decision was simple wanderlust. They needed a change. And as church musicians they already had long experience with living on the margins, at odds with societal expectations. They thought of moving to San Francisco as an experiment, all of us together again in a new kind of commune. They didn't see why *not*.

We had been a family unit for so long. We were a complete choir, and a magical number: seven. They couldn't let us go.

Eventually—a year or so later—with my parents and siblings ensconced in the Turk Street apartment, I moved with a couple of friends into the pretty little flat on Russian Hill, where Howie came to stay every few months, and after that to the cabin in Alaska. I did not live with my parents until I married, or died. I had—I insisted on—a few years to myself. But it was a struggle. In 1982, my grandfather's incipient Alzheimer's disease flared. My parents moved him west along with Great-Uncle Franky to live with them and some of my siblings in a house in Pacifica. And after the money was gone from the sale of the house on Revere Beach, for the rest of their lives my parents skirted the edge of financial doom, a little too old to be working at odd jobs in cities three thousand miles away from where they had lived all their lives, three thousand miles from all their musical contacts. For the rest of their lives, they needed—or threatened to need—rescue from one or another of their children but without ever acknowledging it as rescue.

In 1990, they moved with my sisters Christine and Camille to western Washington state. Camille and Christine had jobs. My parents kept house. My father periodically overdrew Christine's bank account via the ATM card. He had done it once to me during our years in San Francisco, spent my rent, and I'd never let him have my card again after that. When Camille married in 1992 and Christine decided she didn't want to live with our parents anymore, she found and helped them apply for a one-bedroom, rent-subsidized apartment for seniors. It was new, bright, and safe, located in a picturesque Pacific Northwest town, between the mountains and the sea. There was an elevator. Bernadette and her family—who were self-employed—moved to their town to live near them, and my parents saw Bernadette nearly every day. But as time went on, a snit developed with their building manager, who became, in phone conversations I had with my parents, the devil incarnate. *She lives right underneath us. She monitors our every move. We can't drop the soap in the shower without her complaining about the noise. It's torture.*

My parents could charm the birdies out of the trees, if they chose. I wondered why they wouldn't finesse the building manager a little, or at least ignore her, so they could continue to live independently in a place that was clean, safe, and affordable.

Paul and Bernadette bought a house and moved my parents in.

When you're in your forties, you have learned a few things about yourself and your own family dynamics. As Dad and I sat together on the sofa in my TV room, as he half looked at me, not quite asking me if he could live with us, I knew how it would go if he did.

My husband had also grown up in an East Coast, Irish extended family, in apartments in the borough of Queens: a lot of people, a little space, the odd contentious relative in the home. They didn't have a car at all.

But in Howard's family, the response to similar circumstances was a little different. They cultivated independence. Now well up in their seventies, Howard's parents still live in an apartment in Queens. They still have no car. They walk to the local Key Food to get groceries. They bring them home in a two-wheeled shopping cart they keep folded in the front hall; my father-in-law with his bad knees drags them up the concrete stairs in front of the building. They take one, two, sometimes three buses for shopping and doctors' appointments. And when we bring up the idea of moving them out here to live near us, they change the subject.

Sitting on the sofa with my father, I could envision it all. The times we'd ask him, for example, not to drive our cars—my father in his seventies was hard on cars, and our ability to repair or replace them limited—but he'd sneak the keys out of my purse when I wasn't looking and do it anyway. Do it deliberately, even when he had his own brand-new car, knowing it would cause trouble.

Relishing the trouble it would cause. I think, if I'd been single, I would have taken him in. By the age of forty-four, when my dad and I were one-on-one, I'd learned how to fence with him. How to defend what was important to me and relinquish what wasn't. My need for boundaries will never be as fierce as Howard's.

But I wasn't single. If I had said to Howard: *Look, Dad needs a place to live and it's something I want to do*, Howard would have said, *Okay*. But a version of life klieg-lit in front of me that afternoon: the thousand ways my dad would push both our buttons. The times I'd be caught in the middle in my own home, using my dwindling stores of energy in an ongoing struggle to appease and defuse. Feeling cornered in the one place I had always tried to craft a little bit of safety from the world. It was hard enough to broker peace in the extended family for the duration of a holiday dinner.

And there was this: my father loved me, but he also enjoyed watching me tap dance, knowing he had caused it. Something in Dad—something inherently impish but also a little cruel—enjoyed the show at my expense.

No. The answer rose up in me, like bile but also like prayer. My ancestors moaned and shifted in their Massachusetts graves, possibly also in their graves in Ireland and Italy. Maybe my mother's bones rattled too, under her new-dug patch of Pacific Northwest sod.

He still hadn't asked me anything directly. My own spoken answer was also indirect, perhaps also a shade cruel. More about my survival than his.

"I understand, Dad," I said. "I can help you find a little apartment. And I can help you swing it, money-wise, if you need it."

"Ah," he said. His face was careful, neutral. "Okay."

Within two weeks, he was living with Camille and her family.

Camille was philosophic about it. "I understand you didn't feel that Dad could live with you," she said when we talked about it later.

"No," I said. "But I told him I would help him find and maintain his own place to live. He doesn't have to live with you either. I don't think the burden has to fall on you. We could all pitch in and help him in his own place."

"He needs to be with family," she said, a little iron in her voice, and I knew she was right. Though I also thought that much had been sacrificed on the altar of family. And a studio apartment is not a form of torture.

"We're doing fine with him here," she said. "Don't worry

about it. If you can help with the medical side of things, that'll be huge."

There were a few months of grace. He drove his small, gray Suzuki Swift—the new car Bernadette and Paul had bought for him—in the deepening gloom of a Pacific Northwest winter. The gloom pleased him. He loved the climate, the thick forest it produces, the freshness of the rain, much as I do. He made breakfast and lunch dates at greasy spoons with all his children and grandchildren. I saw him every week or so.

In mid-February, Bernadette called to say that she and Camille didn't think he was doing very well. He was short of breath, sleeping all the time, and his feet and legs were both swollen, but the left was larger compared to the right. They thought it was his kidneys, but I knew that both legs would be swollen equally if it was solely his kidneys. This had been going on for several days. They didn't know what to do.

When I pressed him, Dad agreed to see David again. He was having enough trouble breathing that we went via ambulance from clinic to hospital, where he was admitted with blood clots in the femoral veins of both legs, left larger than right, and a probable shower of small clots to his lungs. His chronic kidney failure had worsened again, he was anemic, and his clotting numbers were off. He was also completely disgruntled.

A day later, Kieran, Gabe, and I visited him in his hospital room. He greeted me with the fact that the nephrologist, the kidney doctor, wanted to talk to me; I should ask the nurses to page him. I went down to the nurses' station and set that in motion. When I returned to his room, he launched into a tirade about a CT scan they had tried to do, a survey that would screen for cancer, something I was worried about. He had drunk a little of the contrast medium that would help them get good images but refused to drink it all. They'd done the scan but the quality was poor, and they wanted to repeat it.

He kept saying that there was nothing about the scan that couldn't wait until the following week, when he'd be happy to come back and have it done.

A CT scan is noninvasive, like an x-ray, no needles or scopes or probing fingers. He knew this. And I knew that there was no way he'd return the following week for anything. Also, even if by some éclat he did agree to return, Bernadette or Camille or I would have to spend the lion's share of a day in the car and on ferries, driving him to the hospital and helping him with it.

"How about just getting it all done while you're here?" I said. I was trying for calm and reasonable, but I lost control of the words. They came out in a tiny rush, a fit of temper. "For God's sake, Dad. Why are you making such a huge big deal about a CT scan?" *Huge big FUCKING deal,* is what I wanted to say. But Dad had a roommate who was listening in behind the curtain.

He looked as if I had slapped him. "Be my friend!" he said, seriously aggrieved. His face was bony, crustacean, all large hazel eyes against the bleached white of the sheets. Then his shoulders slumped. "You are just as much of a fanatic as Bernadette and Camille. Medicine is your religion. There's no difference at all. You're nothing but a medical apparatchik. You'll never let it go, no matter what."

Kieran and Gabe were standing behind me, listening closely. Kieran put his hands on my shoulders.

"I think you should leave," Dad said to the boys, the better to berate me without the hulking presence of two somewhat protective young men. They raised their eyebrows, not moving, tacitly asking me what they should do.

"It's okay, guys," I said.

As the door closed behind them, he exploded. "There will never be enough information for these doctors. They will test and test and test. It's all for their information, not for my benefit. None of it is for my benefit. And you're right there with them," he spat.

I did think he was receiving the right care, as much as he'd allow. His clinical picture didn't add up. There were pieces missing, and tests were appropriate.

"They can't treat you unless they find out what's going on," I said, feeling the futility of the words. "Nobody wants to torture you for the hell of it."

"Over the past six months, since last September, *I've* been forced to live with what *you* decided for me," he said then, crossing his arms.

"For chrissake, Dad, that is so unfair. It's not like you were *fine*, pink, fat, and healthy, and I bonked you over the head and dragged you to the doctor. If it ain't broke, I don't believe in fixing it, but you weren't doing *fine* six months ago and you weren't *fine* yesterday when we rode over to the hospital in a medic rig. I wish you wouldn't react to every little need for medical intervention as if it's evidence you're dying. I wish you didn't avoid medical intervention until you are, in fact, dying. I would like it if you'd take care of yourself before you get to death's door."

I was thinking, *I don't want the situation to fall apart so much we can't take care of you.* I was thinking, *I don't want to lose you.* But I didn't say either of those things.

His voice intruded. "Can't you *see* what's wrong with me?" It was an angry, pleading bleat, and it confused me. I had no clue where he was going with this new gambit.

"I'm grieving!" he all but shouted. "That's what happened when my mother died, and that's what's happening now. Once I get past the grief, I'll be fine."

I looked at him. Just talking had made him wheeze and puff. He was a pale bag of bones with eyes. I was beginning to feel like Alice in some malevolent Wonderland, or a player in Sartre's

No Exit version of hell. I took a deep breath to steady myself. It came out as a sigh.

"It's your body and your life, Dad," I said, and I meant it absolutely. "You should do what you want to do about it. It was never my intention to force you to do anything. But if you're waiting for me to *agree* that you're right, it's not going to happen."

Grief didn't cause damaged kidneys from thirteen years of urine backflow. I felt upset at the waste of it. How much discomfort and pain had he endured all those years? He was an intelligent man, and I thought it was flat-out ridiculous. Pigheaded and paranoid. And grief didn't cause huge clots in his femoral veins, though I feel sure it knocked over a physiological domino or two, dominoes that might well have led to all the rest of the mess he was in.

He wanted me to validate his belief that his physical state was solely a reflection of his emotional state, which meant he'd be able to change it at will whenever he decided he had grieved enough. And he wanted me to agree that all medical treatment is needlessly invasive, inhuman, and futile. I would have bought his vision when I was fifteen, and it was my fifteen-year-old self he was reaching for.

But I couldn't pretend I hadn't had this whole other life since then, thirty years' of experience caring for people just like him, people staring right down the gun barrel. I knew where all this was likely to go.

I thought he was receiving reasonably good care, but the system has shortcomings. In the pursuit of health, you are forced to expose the fragile swell of your body to needles and knives, radiation and toxins. And the system isn't geared toward humanistic, tender care, though most of my colleagues struggle against time and staffing limitations to provide as much of that as they can.

Maybe what Dad was saying was he wanted some TLC. That, as we both knew very well, is always the answer to the crossword clue *What RNs dispense.* The trouble is, that clue—with its patronizing implication that TLC is all we provide—never fails to annoy me.

"I think grief is a part of it, Dad, but only a part," I said, after a silence.

"Then we're diametrically opposed, and I suppose that's the end of it," he huffed, folding his arms tight across his chest.

"Look, I'll take myself right out of it. I only wanted to help," I said.

He snorted.

"Do you even want me to speak to the nephrologist?" I felt as if we had paged the guy days ago, but the fact was we were still waiting for him to call back. "I think you should speak for yourself."

"No," he said, mulishly. "I want you to talk to him."

Yeah, and you want to be free to make me your whipping girl for everything, I thought, but I figured I'd do it all the same. In for a penny, in for a pound. Somehow the situation had to move forward.

There was a silence and a lull. Nearly in concert, our heads swiveling at the same time, we turned to the TV set above the bed. Dad had acquired an inexplicable affinity for cooking shows since my mother had died. He had never cooked—his repertoire when I was a child had extended to franks and the odd can of Boston baked beans; he usually burned the franks. And he didn't eat anymore, to speak of. But we watched.

He asked me to rub his back—my gut told me, *No, you don't want to, don't*—but I did it anyway. I felt sick at the state of his shoulders, which had once been thick with muscle that was now completely gone, nothing but jutting bones and skin. He looked like cancer in its end stages, though I told myself he could be anemic, uremic, and in an extreme state of undernourishment, a self-orchestrated starvation in the midst of plenty, all without cancer.

The nephrologist finally called back. He was not my mother's nephrologist; Dad received his care at a city hospital, from a different system. I walked down the long, drab hall to talk to him at the nurses' station, literally dragging my feet. David had e-mailed him about us, told him I was a flight nurse. We talked first about Dad's resistance to procedures. I told him I'd had a fight with Dad, and he volunteered the idea that perhaps I didn't want all that responsibility or to be in that position. I felt absurdly, ridiculously grateful that he understood. He told me he knew he couldn't overcome the years of distrust my father harbored toward the health-care system and that he wanted to care for Dad without torturing him. He had heard my father's theory about it all being a grief reaction—in fact, he had heard all my father's favorite spiels regarding the health-care system, that was obvious—and he said if it was a grief reaction, it was the worst one he had ever seen.

Me too, I thought.

He had asked for a psychiatric consult. *Good luck*, I thought. He said they'd looked for tumors on the CT but didn't find any, and he thought they could dispense with the repeat. He said the urologists would come to consult the following day. I said Dad wouldn't be happy to see them. I said that prostate cancer had been one of my concerns all along, but that Dad had refused to complete the workup during the fall. He said Dad's PSA was 8, and he'd expect it to be higher if prostate cancer was at the root of Dad's problems.

A strange thing, and one of the red flags that sent them on a search for cancer, was that Dad had these huge deep vein clots, but one or more of his clotting factors were abnormal and one of his clotting times—prothrombin time (PT)—was prolonged. There was not a good explanation for this. Normally they would have sent Dad home on Coumadin, an oral blood thinner that prevents further clotting, but Dad's PT acted as if he were already on Coumadin, so that drug was inappropriate. They would want to send him home with daily injections of Lovenox, an anticoagulant that acts on a different part of the clotting cascade. A hematologist would consult.

The last thing he brought up was code status. He asked me how much intervention I thought Dad would want if he should throw a huge clot to his pulmonary artery in the night and try to die. I told him I thought Dad wouldn't want anything—he had said many times he didn't want to be placed on a ventilator under any circumstances, even if it was for something that might improve in a few days. He told me he would talk with Dad and write a Do Not Resuscitate order.

When I went back to Dad's room, I gave him a recap. He was relieved about the CT scan, disappointed that he would need a few more days on IV heparin for the clots in his legs, okay about the possibility of Lovenox at home (I think because when you're talking about what drugs you're going to do at home, it means that there's a chance of your actually going home), and I could tell he didn't want to think about or discuss either the cancer possibility or the no-code status.

So I set him up with his mean, low-salt, renal-diet hospital dinner on the tray table, and left him. Kieran and Gabe put their arms around me on the way out of the hospital.

"Well, that was kind of rough," Kieran said. "Papa acted like a jackass." Kieran had recently turned seventeen. My firstborn, as I was Dad's firstborn.

"You were our love child," Dad used to say to me. "Always so optimistic."

And I would say in my turn that Kieran has always been

good company, right from the first, right from the time he was no more than a blob of goo floating inside my membranes. His steadiness and his excellent humor emanated through the amniotic sac like sound waves.

"It's not *your* fault," Kieran went on as we passed through the swishing double doors in the hospital lobby.

I kissed the tough blond curls above his forehead and wondered what he'd think when the tide and the constellations and the decades turned, and I became Dad and Kieran became me.

The next day when I visited, Howard came along. He crossed his arms, a no-bullshit, New York street-tough gesture, and told my dad, only half joking, that if he yelled at me again, Howard would personally put him on a plane to Texas, where he could live with my sister Christine and her rabbit and go to a hospital in Bush country.

∞

He came home to Camille's basement family room at the end of February, but the downward trajectory was plain. He canceled the one follow-up appointment we had made and snarled at me to leave him alone, and true to my word, I didn't push it. But within a few weeks, he couldn't climb the stairs to the main floor. He left his bed less and less. He ate next to nothing, despite every trick that Camille, our family world-class chef, could dream up. In mid-March, at his request, I took him to Snoqualmie Falls, two hours and a ferry ride away. He wanted to hear the sound of it, he said, the roar and rumble of so much water booming down 270 feet onto the Lower Snoqualmie riverbed. He wanted to feel the mist on his face.

I thought we might be able to talk in the car—my '99 Toyota Sienna CE—maybe even argue, as we always had, but words came hard for both of us. Once we pulled into line in the ferry lot and parked, I waved a ragged Saturday puzzle I had saved. I even offered him the pen. He made a brief effort, but soon closed his eyes, shutting me out. And just like that, staring out at all the other cars waiting to board the ferry on a gray Wednesday noon, I knew for sure he was going to die, though I had no idea why, and I knew our time for talking, which we had always done as easily as breathing, was over. It was already over.

The falls felt like an anticlimax. I wrestled him into a wheelchair and across the footbridge from the parking lot to the viewing area. I didn't know what he wanted—from me, from the falls, from whatever time was left to him, and I wished I could give it to him, whatever it was. If only I could find the Rosetta stone for what it was. But he closed his eyes and listened. The Snoqualmie, swollen with recent spring rains and snowmelt, was at flood stage, running at full voice, in full blood.

On the way home, he shivered, querulous and irritable, and insisted on heat, heat, more heat. I had two blankets wrapped around him and the fan on high, all vents cocked in his direction, feeding febrile blasts from the engine directly at him.

My hands shook on the wheel, my head swam, I felt like throwing up. But when I cracked my driver's-side window, desperate for cool air, he growled at me that he could feel the draft.

∞

At 4:00 a.m. on April 8, Camille's birthday, my father, ignoring Camille's instructions to use the room-to-room monitor to call her if he needed something during the night, got up to get some ice out of the freezer that was about ten steps away. He fell on the way back to bed, and by then, at around ninety pounds, he lacked the strength to scramble to his feet. He lay on the floor, a slab of concrete with a thin veneer of pink and gray wall-to-wall carpet over it, waiting for Camille to rise at six and come down to him. He lay exactly as he fell, like a chalked police outline of himself.

He had been requiring complete care almost around the clock for weeks, and with no end in sight. He had signed a Do Not Resuscitate order for the medics who might respond if called, and we had arranged for hospice care, which was minimal —completely inadequate, in my opinion. A matter of a nurse visiting once a week and managing drugs and supplies by phone, plus an aide who came three times a week for two hours, ostensibly to bathe Dad. There was also a volunteer who came once or twice, a woman who was supposed to help Camille with household tasks but who spent the time venting her own grief about her husband's death. Camille tried to be understanding, but I wanted to strangle her.

Dad wouldn't allow the aide to touch him. He feigned sleep whenever she came. He wanted us, his daughters, to do everything—bathe him, wipe his bottom, change his sheets. Just arranging his pillows the way he wanted was like an hour of Kabuki theater. And by obstructing every movement of the aide, he made sure we did it all. His dentures came in and out of his mouth about twenty times a day, studded with whatever tiny bits of food he had managed to eat. He would hand them to us, still dripping with saliva. I literally gagged each time he did this, and scrabbled for a box of disposable gloves that wasn't there, in that homemade sickroom. The skin on his back was as dry as papyrus; it flaked off, and the itching tormented him. But he wouldn't allow us to put any cream on it, oh no. He wanted us to rub it, *with your hands*, he kept saying. We rubbed it over and over and over and over.

Camille did most of this herself, with the help of her family. The rest of us came over as much as we could to give her breaks. When I took my turn, I tried not to mind the constant back rubs and the ass-wiping, and most of the time I succeeded, but somewhere deep it felt surreal, horrible.

I had to compartmentalize to do it. I have seen so many thousands of bodies now. I've examined them, touched them. Smelled them. Sick people smell bad. They develop rank, organic off-odors on a constant basis. And the certain knowledge that I will be sick and stinky someday too does not make the stench of others any easier to deal with. I've had their blood on my hands, in my eyes, sometimes splattered all over the front of my scrubs or my flight suit. I've brushed their teeth, rinsed their dentures, cleaned stool from under scrotums and from between labia. Suctioned foul yellow mucus from their endotracheal tubes and from deep in their throats.

I've also held their hands, some gnarled, veined, the skin paper-thin—some small, pink, plump with the plenty of childhood. I've stroked their foreheads, brushed their hair, and, if they were babies, kissed their sweet little feet. I know those thousands of bodies. The knowledge is intimate and primal, and it's near total, for the length of a shift. The situation is thrust upon them and on me, and none of us is ever quite ready for it. We just manage with as much good humor as we can muster.

It felt nightmarish to come home to it. I wanted someone else, someone like me, my good twin, perhaps, to wipe the stool from under Dad's scrotum. It didn't help that I thought he was behaving badly. But it should have helped to know he had done it for me, all those many years ago—it should have felt like a fair trade, like a chance to reciprocate for everything he'd given me throughout my life. Not just the food and the shelter, but the singing and the Bach, the love for language and the millions of hours of talk, the doughnuts and the courage to go out and kick ass in any venue I chose, even though I'm a girl. It should have felt good to take care of him. But it didn't.

Camille usually rose at six. However, on her birthday, for the one and only time, while Dad was dying in her basement, she slept until eight. It was her version of kicking up her heels for the occasion. But that meant Dad spent four hours instead of two staring in the dark at the carpet pattern, freezing on a concrete slab.

When I arrived at ten to take over for her so she could go out for what I hoped would be a festive birthday lunch with her family, the whole household was in an uproar.

"I feel so bad," she said upstairs in her kitchen, her husband and sons crowded around. She was literally wringing her hands. "He lay there for so many hours. I can't believe it. The one time I slept late."

When she had finally come down to the basement and found him, he had screamed at her for neglecting him, she told me. She looked so upset—so exhausted and spent, her freckles standing out in stark relief against her pallor—that I was suddenly angry on her behalf. Unlike Camille, I am in touch with my inner bitch. For better or worse.

"First of all," I said, "I submit to you that ice for his glass is not of prime importance in the middle of the night."

"I know," she said, "but it's so awful to think about him lying there."

"And you told him what to do. You told him to call."

"That's true," she said.

"Well, he didn't do it. I know he's sick, and I hate the idea of him lying on the floor all that time as much as you do, but here's the thing: he's still a person, an adult who makes choices. He's a stubborn old geezer, and he does whatever the fuck he wants."

I heard Camille's husband, Kevin, who had a real affection for Dad and was very patient with him, snort a laugh. I believe Kevin's family is likewise full of Norwegian/Irish old geezers who do whatever *they* want.

I saw Camille bite back a small grin and felt encouraged.

"This time, he chose to ignore you, and it bit him in the ass. Next time, I bet he'll call."

After I ushered them all out the door toward lunch, I girded my loins and descended the stairs. Dad looked contrite from his hospital bed in the corner. Resilience was his strong suit. He had already rebounded.

"I shouldn't have yelled at her," he told me. "It was my own fault."

"Oh, Dad," I sighed. "Just call her next time."

"I don't want to bother them while they're sleeping," he said.

"We can put a cooler with some ice in it on your table at night," I said.

Chickie and Kathy arrived for a visit in mid-April, and we knew it would be the last. Easter came in late April, and we all spent it at Camille's together. Dad was animated that day. His laughter was startling in his skeletal face, booming out, his grin huge, goofy, and toothless, still somehow vital.

Camille and I had ongoing talks about how long it might take. Round-the-clock care is inhuman for the caregiver. People can yap all they want about the altruism of it, and none of us wanted him to die in a SNF, pronounced "sniff," a skilled-nursing facility, but you can't keep up that level of care alone at home forever. Realistically, I feel people can do it for a week, maybe two. I know how exhausted I am after a twelve-hour shift of it. The longer it goes on, the more it bankrupts the caregiver. Short of quitting my job, which I was not at liberty to do, I couldn't take over for Camille. But he had been bed-bound since March, and it was exacting a huge toll.

And I didn't know how much longer it would take. The

human body is so tough, so resilient. True, he weighed about eighty pounds. True, he wasn't eating anything. But he was still drinking a little root beer, a little water. Urine still drained into the bag through the Foley. He refused pain meds, sipped at Johnnie Walker Red all day instead. This was weird. He had been a teetotaler for most of his life, until he'd gotten sick. Until he started self-medicating, as we say in the trade.

I told Camille that if it was too much, I would arrange for care in a SNF. I told her that had I been in her shoes, I would already have reached my limit. I told her I would be the bad guy; I'd tell him he had to go. *Not yet*, she said, *not yet*.

Camille, Bernadette, and I all began to notice he avoided the topic of death. He talked instead as if he were getting better, as if his current condition were just a little detour. He told Chickie and Kathy he was under the care of a doctor, and he was, but for comfort care, the only care he'd accept. We did not know how to handle this. It seemed cruel to remove hope. Hope is an odd thing. Sometimes it honestly is a saving grace. And we didn't even know what was wrong with Dad. None of the things we knew about were fatal in and of themselves. I thought it would be wrong, philosophically, to place him on death row in my mind and abandon him there with no hope of reprieve. But the reality was: weaker and weaker, thinner and thinner. The reality was he refused treatment.

"I'm afraid he's going to turn into one of those people who's stuck between life and death, like the people in nursing homes who go on for years," Camille said, and I understood the worry. A long time ago, as nurses' aides, both Camille and I had cared for those people. Silent and withered, their eyes were filmy with some perpetual, impenetrable twilight. Their limbs were so contracted and immobile that they flipped over all of a piece, as unwieldy as a small dining table, when we turned them in bed from one side to the other.

But I shook my head. "One of these days, sometime soon, he's going to ask me point-blank if he's dying," I said to Camille. "I know he will. And I'm not going to lie to him."

∾

It came on May 2, to be exact.

"I want to know from you what my clinical prognosis is." He loosed the question at me the second I approached the bed.

My stomach rolled up into a tiny little ball, like a hedgehog in hiding. *Oh nae, lassie*, it said, a stomach with a Scottish accent. I felt nauseated. But if I didn't exactly leap into the breach, I did at least dip a cautious toe into it.

"You're not doing very well, Dad."

He didn't buy the equivocation. "No!" he said, agitated and intense. His furry white brows gathered like thunderheads. "I want to know what my clinical prognosis is. Do you think I'm dying?"

In my mind, I took a deep breath. In reality, I'm sure I was hyperventilating. *Is it possible to feel heartbroken and sick of his crap at the same time?* I wondered.

"Yes, Dad, I think you're dying."

There was a shocked and angry silence from him, almost a nonverbal howl, and I thought, *You have got to be shitting me, how did it come to this*, but I pressed on.

"You're worse every time I see you. You've lost thirty more pounds; you've lost all your muscle. You're weaker. You're able to do less and less. You can't turn over in bed by yourself. You have a bedsore. You're . . . *worse every time*," I repeated, lamely. Desperately.

"I can't tell that," he huffed.

"I know—maybe it's hard to tell because you're living it minute by minute—but I come every week and I see the changes."

Maybe it's hard to tell? Four weeks ago you became the poster boy for the Life Alert Emergency Response: "Help, I've fallen and I can't get up!"

Once upon a time I would have been able to share the running commentary in my head with him. I wish now that I had. He might actually have laughed. Even then.

He shrugged. "So what is your clinical opinion and prognosis?"

I had no idea what to say or where to start. "Well, as far as I can tell, it's from renal failure," I began. *Or cancer? Starvation? You didn't exactly cooperate with the workup.*

"Are the kidneys gone, dead?" he all but roared.

"Let me sit down," I said. I pulled up a chair. We kept the room hot—eighty-five degrees, it felt like. I sat on my (*Stop that, not now!*) trembling hands.

"No, Dad, they're not dead completely."

He grunted in satisfaction. *See?* he seemed to be saying. *How can you say I'm dying?*

"They make urine, but as far as I can tell, from the last tests you had, which were three months ago now, they don't get rid of waste products very well. I think your mind is fine (*Fine?*) and from what I can see, your spirit is alive and looking ahead (*?*), but your body doesn't seem to be cooperating at all. It seems to be going the other way. The wrong way."

"So you're just waiting for me to die?" He sounded hurt, disbelieving, spitting mad. "I'm going to die today?" he asked, sarcastically.

"I don't know what's in store for you, Dad. I can only tell you what I see."

Silence.

After a while, I asked him if there was anything I could get for him.

"What's the use of getting anything for me?" He sounded

as furious and hurt as an eighty-pound sentient skeleton can sound.

"Why are you angry with me, Dad?"

"Guess."

"I'm not guessing anything," I said, the inner bitch rising up in protest. "You'll just have to tell me why you're so mad."

He patted his chest and breathed with difficulty for a moment or two.

"Child of my heart," he said finally. "Presenting me with such hopelessness."

With a corner of my mind, I thought, *You are such an Irish drama king.* With another corner, I thought, *You are so unfair.* But the rest of me had no heart at all for the game, if that's what it was.

"Not hopelessness, Dad," I said. "Honesty. You asked me to tell you. I'm just trying to be honest." *And it's uphill work.*

"You don't have to be so brutal about it," he said, then either fell asleep or feigned it.

While he slept, or feigned sleep, I did wonder just how brutal I was. I still don't have any answer. Later that same day, I called Julie—my highly irreverent friend Julie, she who rides from Seattle to Portland with us every summer—and told her about this conversation. She is a pediatric nurse-practitioner; we worked in the PICU together for years. She doesn't have much tolerance for bullshit, parental or otherwise. She said, "I think it might be time to smother him with a pillow."

After a while, he woke up. He said, "It's a nice day."

This was an olive branch.

"I don't *want* you to die, Dad," I said, and sighed.

To this, there was no response. He closed his eyes again. He shut me out.

A few minutes later, after he either woke or pretended to

wake, he asked for a back rub, which I provided. He lightened the mood a bit. I offered a beer; he accepted.

"*La vie . . .*," he toasted, lifting the glass.

"Skoal," I said. I felt like guzzling the whole thing. Plus some scotch.

After a while I asked, "What do you think about down here all the time, Dad?"

He hesitated, as if he might not want to tell me, but then he did.

"Snatches of songs," he said.

"Snatches of songs!" I don't know what I expected, but it wasn't that. "Well, I guess that's not so surprising." *You are a musician, after all.* "Which songs?"

"Love songs," he said after a bit, and he sang a line from Three Dog Night's "An Old Fashioned Love Song." Even in extremis, only half trying, his bel canto tenor still had a vital hook in it.

"Hey, *Harmony,* 1971." I laughed. That was the second album I bought as a teenager. It was terrible, of course. One of those stinkers you will have forever in your vinyl collection. I remember that Dad was with me when I bought it, at the mall in Shrewsbury, Massachusetts, in the record store on the upper level. I remember that he offered to buy me Bach instead: Glenn Gould, the French and English suites. A much better value for the long term. But I declined. At that time, at age thirteen, I wanted more than anything to shake the dust of classical music off my feet.

After a while I added, "Somebody had to bring rock and roll into the house, Dad . . . it might as well have been me." *Eve tempts Adam in the Garden of Eden,* I thought.

"It's a shame," he said primly, as though he had been thinking the very same thing.

After a minute or two he added, " 'Waiting for the *Robert E. Lee* . . .' " Another song.

"I don't remember 'The *Robert E. Lee*,' Dad," I said.

"The levee." He panted and spat into a sheet of paper towel. I waited.

A brief Web search informed me, years later, that "Waiting for the *Robert E. Lee*" was a song from the movie *Babes on Broadway*. Judy Garland, Mickey Rooney. The lyrics were terrible, a long way from his usual musical territory—but my dad, I think, was a secret fan of Judy Garland's. He had a few of her albums in his collection. And he would have been fourteen in 1941, the year the movie was released. Two years away from meeting my mother.

In his room, at the other end of his life, I was poised for enlightenment.

"People waiting on the levee for the ship to come in," he said, as if that explained everything.

He closed his eyes again. I could tell it was real this time. Finally, he woke and told me, "I'm going to keep falling asleep on you." I asked him if he wanted to sleep for a while, because if he did, I'd go up and clean Camille's kitchen for her. He agreed.

I kissed the top of his head.

"I love you, Dad," I offered.

"I know it," he accepted.

∾

He died four days later, on May 6. Just shy of eleven months after my mother. I did not talk to him again. I was on the opposite side of Puget Sound when he took a final wrong turn—stopped talking, stopped thinking, finally stopped breathing. There was too much open water between us for me to make it to his bedside before the end.

But then, there's this: As I worked on telling this tale, right after I wrote down the bones of our final conversation, I took a break to do the *New York Times* crossword. Another rainy winter dusk was falling here in the Pacific Northwest; it softened, blurred, and finally erased the cedars and hemlocks that peer into the window above my desk. I did not have the *New York Times* in hand; I did it via the Web for the first time ever, surprised to see that my Sunday-only subscription to the paper entitled me to a premium crossword subscription online. I much prefer the hard copy; you can't, after all, save an online crossword for later use in an automobile or a waiting room.

It was a Thursday in January 2008, and there was a new puzzle, but each day they also offer a classic puzzle from the archives, and I chose that to start with. The archives go back years and years; perhaps it was a puzzle from the Eugene T. Maleska era. I'll never know for sure, because I clicked it closed when I finished it and lost it forever. But nevertheless, for however brief a moment, there it was. In watery blue computer light, shining forth in the dark, a clue:

—"Waiting for the *Robert E. Lee*" film.

Chapter Eleven

Night Vision

It's November now in the Pacific Northwest, and dark comes early. The dregs of daylight drain fast, and sometimes I plan to do a forty-five-minute ride after a day at the desk but miss the window of opportunity. I'm not one of those who can drop down pitch-black hills on a bike with a tiny headlamp, on a wing and a prayer. I don't perceive light the way I used to, particularly in my left eye, where the nerve has been damaged and there's a hole in the world, a spot that starts out the size of a peppercorn but grows, as my body temperature rises, to the shape of a kidney bean. In the dark at thirty-five miles an hour, I'd be flying blind.

But I need my hit of exercise, so instead I walk the roads here at night. At three or four miles an hour, I won't get the same high-voltage jolt of adrenaline, the same pure endorphin rush I get on my bike. I won't run my heart rate up to 150. But neither will I miss the branch blown down in the road, the patch of deep gravel, the lump of newspaper in the street.

It's damp and cold in November, often raining. There aren't any sidewalks or streetlamps, just houses behind trees, a few glimmers of living room light. As a driver, I know how invisible pedestrians can be alongside the roads here. As a flight nurse who has lifted from the scenes of hundreds of motor vehicle accidents, from plenty of highways and byways, I know just how a body looks after it's been bucked into the air by two tons of

SUV. I wear my reflective yellow biking jacket; I clip a strobing red light to my back and carry a bright flashlight.

But the flow of traffic on this island depends on boatloads of commuters disgorged every fifty minutes. It isn't constant. There are long minutes when I switch off my flashlight, long minutes with no traffic at all, when I'm alone with a ribbon of road and the most recent rain's runoff gurgling in the drainage ditches that run by the side of every road around here. Alone with the damp smell of mud, of cedars and firs. Alone with the night sky and my own damaged night vision.

∽

The first clear omen was that long-ago autumn evening, the evening I cried in front of my apartment building after running errands in our old Chevy, daunted by three flights of stairs and twelve-pound newborn Gabe. I was thirty years old. And the postpartum period is a classic time for a multiple sclerosis exacerbation, I've since learned. The hormonal changes of pregnancy appear to decrease the episodes of inflammation that destroy myelin. Myelin is the fatty insulation surrounding nerve fibers in the brain and spinal cord; it's the white matter in the white-matter/gray-matter equation of the brain. But if pregnancy is protective in MS, the postpartum period leaves you vulnerable.

What I know now: both intrinsic (body) heat and extrinsic (ambient) heat can make MS symptoms worse until something comes along to cool you down. Physically worse, though it's easy enough to feel like some kind of hothouse flower, to think it's all in your head. Heat slows impulses across damaged nerves. If you have MS, your actual physical performance might well degrade when you're warm from exercise, from fever, when it's eighty in the summer. If you're on the milder end of the MS spectrum, you can come in from a strenuous bike ride, take a hot shower, and then have to scoot up the stairs on your ass, your legs a little too rubbery to hold you. This *will* make you feel crazy.

Maybe the car heater was on a little too high that evening as I drove home from the mall. And maybe the cutting ocean wind cooled me as I labored to extract Gabe from the car seat. But here's the dual-edged irony, poised over all my days since. It's both how I'm lucky and the monkey on my back. There was no absolute. No final *I can't*. I climbed the stairs. I didn't drop Gabe. I didn't have to call 911. I didn't even have to call my husband to bail me out. So what if my back ached with spasms like a bad tooth as I climbed and for hours afterward; so what if I needed to recover from my own stairs as if from an illness. And that lack of an absolute, *I can do it when I try*, leads to a corollary: *I'm not trying hard enough.*

∞

In the early part of my life, when I was an arrogant young thing, I hardly ever looked up. The stars in Boston were cold, few, and distant, the lights of the city too bright. But in 1994, when I was thirty-five, I floated down the Colorado River in a sixteen-foot raft through Grand Canyon. It was a private trip; Rob was a guide on the Colorado before life moved him downstream. Before he married Lori, who ten years later became my coworker and friend in an intensive-care nursery in California, before he fathered a couple of girls, earned an MBA, and learned to navigate the waters of corporate life with what I imagine is the same flair, the same combination of curiosity and balls and intelligent, intuitive analysis that kept him out of holes on the river.

Prior to the Grand Canyon trip, Rob ran two of the guys in the planned party of sixteen down the American River and trained them to row white water. But he was still one man short of a full complement of oarsmen. On a night shift in the intensive-care nursery, Lori and I hatched a plan. Thinking of the mass of my husband's biceps and his love for any body of water, I volunteered Howard to be one of the boatmen on the Colorado. "He's strong and smart," I told Lori, by way of a rowing résumé. To that point, the sum total of Howard's experience in boats amounted to one half-day trip as a passenger down a river in Pennsylvania, a river with a couple of middling rapids. That, and riding the Staten Island ferry in his native New York.

But somehow, rowing eight hours a day on the Colorado in June of 1994, Rob—and Howard, Jon, Brian, and Greg—pulled it off. They rowed the big water in Grand Canyon: Hance and Sockdolager, Crystal and Lava Falls. Huge rapids—8, 9, 10, 10 plus on a rating scale of 1 to 10. Nobody died. Howard rowed like hell, training with Rob the first week, running his own boat the second. He burned enough calories that even though he has insulin-dependent diabetes, he was able to eat pound bags of M&M's and never turn a blood glucose above 120.

But it's the nights I want to remember now, nights lying next to the river. It's the shrieking antediluvian hiss of cicadas in the evening, the infinite, implacable sound of water over rock that infiltrated my dreams. I threw out my sleeping bag next to a wall of Vishnu schist that is 1.7 billion years old, lay on my back on sand that gave up the relentless desert heat of the day a little at a time. I stared up into a prehistoric night, far from any city, cut by the absolute black of the canyon rims. The sky above the canyon was a narrow swath, loaded with stars.

I remember the spill of the Milky Way; I think I saw the Dippers, Big and Little. I *know* I felt my place in the order of the universe, the sure knowledge that I'm not even a flash in the pan. Not even a mote in the eye of God. I still believed in God then. During the day, on some of the nastier rapids, I prayed. You have to reach down deep to find the goods to row the Colorado, and with the exception of Rob and his brother Jon, our boatmen didn't have experience on their side. I prayed that Howie and Rob and the boys were strong enough and smart enough. But under the night sky of the canyon, prayer seemed beside the point. I understood I was a nanosecond, a pictogram, a tiny arc across a single synapse. That at most I could hope to be a mote of Vishnu schist someday. The thought was—is—strangely comforting. A relief.

Yet the feature of that sky that I remember best was a faint pinprick, fainter than the lowest magnitude of stars, distinguishable only by its speed. I haven't seen it since—I'm a denizen of cities and suburbs, polluted by light. It sailed across the canyon sky in a matter of a few minutes, an undignified human tumble across the lower heavens. A satellite.

∞

I'm not trying hard enough. That's a concept I still struggle with, twenty years after that moment in front of my building, the moment that only in retrospect was a watershed for me. There were thirteen years between that evening and diagnosis in late 2001—years haunted by fatigue that was omnipresent and occasionally flared to devastating (*But I'm working nights*), with tense, spastic muscles aching like they do with flu (*For chrissake, do I have hidden psychic traumas, or am I coming down with something again?*), toes that caught on linoleum and hands that knocked things over (*Shit, I'm clumsy!*). Memory lapses I was decades too young for; dizziness that made the world rock on its keel for a while, several times a day. But significant as the whole picture is in the aggregate, no single symptom was severe enough or persistent enough to raise a red flag. So on every one of those days, I told myself it was imaginary. I ragged on myself for some self-perceived lack—of assertiveness or endurance, of discipline or drive.

Yet I raised two boys from babyhood to adolescence in those years. Between bouts of falling off the exercise wagon, I ran, I swam, I biked; I pressed a fair amount of weight at the gym. I worked full-time in frantic, pressured settings—in intensive-care nurseries, pediatric intensive-care units, labor-and-delivery units. At brutal accident scenes and tiny referring hospitals with few resources. In the air and on the ground. And under it all a half-conscious notion: *You can't be sick and do all that.*

We tend, as a culture and even as health-care providers, to think of disability in terms of either/or, black or white, can or can't. When it's largely invisible, when some days you can do things easily, and some days you can do them with a big effort, and some days, in spite of bringing every personal resource to bear, you can't do anything at all, what then? It doesn't feel like disability. It just feels like failure.

Several times a week for five years, I climbed into the back of the helicopter—the Agusta A109 Mark II—and took off into the night sky. We never knew what we were going to face. Maybe an unconscious twenty-five-year-old with a sucking chest wound by the side of a rural road, or a kind old man in a suburban ER with an evolving heart attack, pumped full of nitroglycerin. Sometimes a premature baby at an outlying hospital and no pediatrician for a hundred miles. That meant that we—pilot and two nurses—had to wrestle the 250-pound transport Isolette into the Agusta by the light of Mini Mags held in our teeth. There was grunting and swearing involved.

But the night does its work, regardless. There's expansion

in the night. No limits. It filled every window of the aircraft, and I rode it, in royal blue Nomex with my boots up on the stretcher platform. I was grubby, usually spent, sometimes bitter about being wrenched from sleep, but the night was out there anyway, omnipresent. Mountains receded into it; the ocean became a void under it.

On the outbound leg, I'd try to gather myself for the work ahead as we dodged storm cells and cloud banks in fall and winter, as we searched for safe passage into a black hole of a landing zone where a patient waited, a landing zone ringed by trees and power lines and fences that were all the color of night. We'd slip through 1,500 feet of wee-hour haze in summer. They were soft, humid nights that felt like love in spite of our bloody circumstances, nights that rendered early, rosy dawns.

On the inbound leg, my partner and I would sometimes sweat bullets under a single pale dome lamp, our attention lasered inward on somebody sick, somebody circling the drain, somebody trying too hard to go toward the light. Outside, the night kept watch.

The stars whistled past, and not only stars. Sometimes, staring at a bright spot on a dark horizon, I couldn't tell if it was star or aircraft. I'd strain toward it, searching for red or green, for the blink and flash that would tell me it was human, not cosmic.

Over time, I had flare-up after flare-up, and each one lingered for a couple of months. I had multiple courses of intravenous steroids that improved the MS symptoms but left me feeling dizzy for weeks. Dizzy and depressed, like the world was flat and tasteless, like I was looking at my life through the wrong end of a telescope. I developed an intermittent tremor. Its severity shocked me at times, particularly when I was hot. My sense of balance became more impaired. My right foot went numb to the ankle with any sort of activity. My bladder started acting cranky. I could sort of *correct* for it all most of the time, but it took more and more energy to do that.

Adrenaline and camaraderie kept me going at work. Conditioning increases your energy if you have MS, within limits, and I exercised every day. The pounding of running made me spasm into a pretzel shape; swimming at a public pool—the scheduled lap swim, drying off, redoing my hair—was too much work. Biking in the cool northwest air became my sport of choice.

But at home, even on my fourth day off, I was sleeping on the sofa for much of the rest of the time. I didn't get into bed. That would have been throwing in the towel. If I slept on the sofa, the all-day nap didn't really count—I could trick myself into thinking my fatigue wasn't that bad. But I was too tired to get up for a drink of water when I was thirsty. Too tired to put in a load of laundry, oversee my sons' homework. I tried to goad myself into more productivity—*Suck it up*—but it didn't work. You can pull yourself up by your bootstraps for a hell of a long time, I was learning, but not every day for the rest of your life.

And there were the shots of high-dose interferon beta-1a I gave myself three times a week, designed to suppress my immune system, or at least the part of it that destroys myelin. You're supposed to take it at night before bed, to minimize the side effects, which are described as "flu-like symptoms." But one night, I forgot. I took it when I woke up at five in the morning instead, before I left for a twenty-four-hour helicopter shift at our northern suburban base, a long drive from home. Mistake. By the time I got to work, my whole body ached so much that even the hair follicles in my scalp hurt.

My partner that Thursday was one of my favorite people

to fly with. Originally from Montana, she'd been a flight nurse forever—fifteen years at least. Huge blue eyes, could think on her feet, arms like she swam the two-hundred-meter butterfly. Irreverent. Like others in our cohesive little organization of health professionals, she knew my story of MS and interferon. She took a look at me and said, "You wanna go home, honey?"

"No," I said. Not after driving two hours to get there. "Though this *is* like a fucking bout of Ebola," I added, and she laughed.

I knew if I ate 800 milligrams of Advil and slept for a while, it'd get better. I thought that if worst came to worst, and a flight came along in the interim, I'd manage to deal. If you're busy enough, a flight is an out-of-body experience.

"I'll check the aircraft, then," she said. "You get a little shut-eye, doll."

I fell under the covers in my bedroom in our hangar quarters, wearing all my clothes and shivering like I was septic. I should have gone home, of course, but the flight gods held off. I woke up at eleven that morning, still aching like a mother-fucker. Took some more Advil, let sleep swallow me again. At three in the afternoon, I finally surfaced. The aches weren't completely gone, but my hair didn't hurt. It *was* manageable. I did a little happy dance at the improvement. I drank a little water, ate a little toast.

At 3:45 p.m., the pagers beeped for a field response sixty miles away. A worried medic; a two-year-old, obtunded, nearly unconscious. She had an overwhelming infection—she was sep-tic, the real thing. Her blood pressure was starting to crash and burn; my partner and I went to work. And right after we landed her, with a better blood pressure, at the ER of the children's hospital, there was a guy on a back road somewhere, T-boned in his small utility pickup by some other, bigger vehicle. A shattered pelvis. We stabilized it with a sheet pulled tight around his hips, resuscitated him with fluid while we flew him to the trauma center. We relieved his pain with morphine.

"The smell of Jet A in the afternoon." I laughed as we hopped out of the helicopter while the pilot powered it down back at quarters. "I love it."

"Amen, sister," she said, slapping my hand, high-five.

I was feeling *fine*. People with real problems we could do something about. A cosmos of training and experience—thirty whirling years—that I could bring to bear on every single flight. A gorgeous, sunny afternoon and hundreds of miles of open sky. Rock and roll, motherfucker! I felt way more than fine—I felt like I was going to live forever. I just couldn't make it last.

∞

I took medical leave. My friends—my partners—donated vacation hours to me by the hundreds. I've always worked for the money, honey, not the love of it. The words *long-term disability* and *Social Security* became a part of my lexicon. But the drabness and hopelessness of the Social Security office—any Social Security office, anywhere—gives you the urge to bury a knife in your own neck (as a depressed patient of mine once did—amazingly enough, he missed every single vital structure and went home within a day). It's no mean feat to pass the review for Social Security disability insurance; lots of people are denied. I submitted hundreds of pages of documentation to support my claim. But when I told Howie, nine months into my leave, that my SSDI application had been approved, I burst into tears.

Despite SSDI and private disability insurance, outgo exceeded income. Health insurance alone, which will never be a luxury again, cost nearly eight hundred dollars per month when my husband put me on his plan.

I went to bed in my own home every single night, though. I slept whenever I needed to, which was all the time, at first. If I had a flare-up and lost two weeks to worsening symptoms or steroids, no one had to fill my shifts at time and a half or double time. I didn't have to brace my arm against tremor to start an IV or slip a tube into a trachea; I didn't have to sling a heavy stretcher around a muddy, potholed field trying to right myself through dizziness. I didn't have to carry eighty pounds through the body aches of interferon and spasticity. I could go to the bathroom five times an hour if my bladder insisted on it. It was all such a relief.

And I began—slowly, slowly, slowly—to feel less exhausted. At first, I'd planned to take a year off, try to recover whatever health I could, then return to work. But the thought of taking all that up again—all those burdens—raised a faint flutter of panic. And I had seen my neurologist one month after I stopped working. Her words stuck with me.

"How do you feel?" she had asked. "Your MRI has a few more lesions. Your neuro exam—kind of plus/minus. But you *look* better."

"I feel better," I admitted. "Less fatigued. I didn't know it was possible. I've felt exhausted for so long I thought it was just my baseline. But I still tire so easily. A couple hours of activity and I'm cooked."

My neurologist is neat, exact, about ten years younger than I am. Sometimes that makes me feel world-weary and ancient. But she's awesome, in her way. Time is brain in MS—the earlier immunomodulatory treatment begins, the more function is likely to be preserved—and she's aggressive with the disease process, collaborative and supportive with me. But it can't be easy. Her practice is all MS, and it is a permanent, ultimately progressive disease. Always a net loss for her patients, or at best, treading water—month after month, year after year. Symptoms, visible and invisible, that range from annoying to devastating, and the best available treatments for those symptoms so stop-gap and imperfect. Problems you can manage a bit, but never solve.

She eyed me through her chic little smart-girl glasses.

"You've bounced back this much," she said, gesturing knee-high. "With more time, who knows? You might come to here," she continued, marking an imaginary line at her waist. "Maybe even further.

"It's certainly not my place to say you *can't* ever work again. You have to decide what quality of life means to you. Some people derive most of it from their work. But you've been dealt a hand you didn't ask for. I think you should consider *not* going back."

It was a relief to feel understood. We did the paperwork as if for a permanent retirement, but inside, where it counts, I tabled the decision. At the one-year mark, I had a relapse, and it took a few months to recover. My boss filled my position. It hurt. At the eighteen-month mark, I flared up again. Still, between relapses my baseline was getting better and better all the time, my energy less fleeting, less fragile. I probed the envelope of fatigue. I began to understand that my energy was a finite resource, began to learn what would increase it, what would deplete it. I needed seven hours or more of sleep every night; that was the first thing. If I got six and a half, the blinding, over-whelming exhaustion came right back.

I needed exercise every single day, but it cut two ways. It stretches the point for me to call myself an athlete, but to the extent that I'm active, I'm about distance and endurance. All slow-twitch muscle. My lone athletic asset has always been that I can keep it up—enjoy keeping it up—long past the time when most sensible people would quit for the day. MS hasn't changed that yet, not completely, but there is a limit. A point in every workout, and it shifts every day, at which the humoral forces of destruction in my brain and spinal cord begin to ramp up.

Outside of the fatigue, my neuro symptoms waxed and waned, as they do in MS. Overall, being well rested, I had longer stretches with fewer problems. On good days, days I rode fifty hilly miles, it felt like cheating to be on disability. On bad days, I lay on the sofa with my hands shaking and the world spinning, grateful I wasn't in the air.

But the Agusta never left me alone. Several times a week the sound of the aircraft overhead hooked me from sleep, deep in the night. It nailed me coming and going, outbound and inbound on flights to the peninsula. The sound was—still is— a deep, insistent, vibratory drone. The drone of two big jet engines across half a mile of space. It started low and grew until it dwarfed my bedroom. Once you've heard the Agusta, you can't mistake it for anything else.

It suffused my dreams, made them anxious and uneasy. I dreamed over and over again that the pager had gone off but I couldn't find my flight suit or my helmet. I couldn't find my boots. I dreamed of flights in their entirety, down to the last detail, down to the baby's weight in kilograms, the vital sign numbers, and the antibiotics that were hung, but I was always only a bystander. I could never get off the ground in my dreams; something always interfered.

At the peak of the droning, if I was awake and not dreaming, I'd catch a glimpse of the blinking streak, a streak that contained at least three souls, all of them friends. My bedroom window could frame it for only an instant.

∞

I almost always have the road to myself as I warm to a walking rhythm, as I tromp past Point Monroe and along Port Madison, trailed everywhere I go by the night sky. The moon, if there is one, lingers over Kane Cemetery. Sometimes I loop through that tiny graveyard that overlooks the sea, halfway down the hill on Lafayette. I like the dead to know I remember them, even though they're not my dead. My parents are buried forty miles from here, and I used to fly over their graves several times a week, far more often than I'll ever manage to go there in my car. I was able to fix on them from 1,500 feet because of the middle school that lies next to the cemetery. Their graves are near the fence that divides graveyard from schoolyard, about halfway between the road and the white statue of the Virgin Mary. When I prepared myself for a flyby, when I realized they were in our flight path, when I took my bearings, sought them out, and watched as their burial place slid down my window, under my boots on the floor of the helicopter cabin, and out into our slipstream, it felt right. It felt like ritual. Like respect.

As I walk, the sky seems close. But the city is right across the water, fewer than nine miles to the east, and there are so often clouds. Stars are insignificant here. Aircraft take primacy. There's a half-mile stretch at Port Madison with a clear view to the north, and as I pass along the shoreline there, warm enough now to shed my jacket even in November, I usually see a dozen or more crisscrossing the sound. They wink their way toward Whidbey or Camano islands, Snohomish or Jefferson counties. I can follow them in my mind to a landing zone in a park on Whidbey, where at eleven one Friday night, my partner and I picked up a man my age in respiratory distress after transplantation. I can still see the man. Salt-and-pepper hair, alert, and sweet-natured despite his long list of medical problems. Maybe because of them—the patience they can teach you. I can see the rig and the medics, the shrubbery around the perimeter of the park, and the wet gravel drive. I can see the tall trees that are ever present in this area, this temperate rain forest overlaid by city and suburb. Our guy had received multiple organ transplants, but I've lost my grip on which ones. Liver and kidney? Heart and lung?

For every flashing light up there, there's a different LZ, another story, another undignified human tumble. The sky, hardboiled and helicoptered, will never let me go, not completely. Its absence is conspicuous in the tiny clinic exam room—windowless—where I mainline IV steroids with each significant flare-up. But it follows me whenever I ride, when I push myself faster and further, straddling the line between endurance and destruction. November dusk trails me into the gym as I work lats and biceps, triceps and pecs, as I brace myself against tremor to leg press 290, 300, 310 pounds, thinking of the 150-, 250-, 300-pound patients that are out there, waiting for a stretcher. For someone's stretcher, if not for mine. The early evening sky glows small in the gym window, immense out here on this rain-slick road, where Port Madison's tide surges toward the open sea. It's bright with celestial bodies ancient and new, bodies from both the upper and lower reaches of heaven.

Chapter Twelve

Out There in the Deep

#4

The call came at about 2215 on September 29, 2005, nearly two years into my medical leave. The voice on the phone belonged to Tom, the colleague whose name was above mine on the phone tree, and I was glad to understand that my name still appeared on the phone tree. He told my son it was urgent, and Gabe brought the phone into my bedroom. I was almost but not quite asleep.

The essence of the message was this: one of our helicopters was fifty minutes overdue.

Fifty minutes. Forever.

At 2104, the crew—two nurses and pilot—had lifted off the hospital helipad. They had delivered a patient and were bound for quarters at Arlington, our northern suburban base. It was a trip I had made hundreds of times. It usually took about fifteen to twenty minutes.

What we commonly referred to as a flight—the transport of a patient from a prehospital site or from a referring hospital to a receiving hospital—was actually a mission composed of at least three flights, three separate takeoffs and landings. There was the outbound leg to the accident scene or the referring hospital, the inbound leg to the receiving hospital with the patient onboard, and the return-to-quarters leg for the crew.

I thought of this last as the dead leg of a flight or, sometimes, as the latte leg, if I was able to score at the coffee kiosk before we took off. I kept a twenty-dollar bill in a small zippered pocket over my left biceps, just for that purpose. This part of the mission was a relief, a few minutes to put my feet up on the stretcher platform and sightsee out the window. A time to decompress in the small womb of the cabin, lulled by vibration—the roar of the engines muted to a hum by my helmet. The official term for the dead leg is a *14 CFR Part 91 positioning flight.*

The last radar return was recorded at 2112, near Edmonds. Shortly thereafter, there were 911 calls from the Edmonds area. They all reported the same thing: the sound of a helicopter overhead, followed by the sound of an explosion. I envisioned flames, but the evidence had all been auditory. Nobody had seen anything.

I knew right then they were dead. If they weren't dead, if the 911 calls were a fluke, they'd have radioed or called. If any of the three of them had an intact finger to push a button, they'd have been in touch.

I climbed out of bed, clad only in the soft old T-shirt I wear for pajamas.

"Who's on it?" I asked.

The question wasn't whether friends were on it. That was a given. The question carried a different kind of mortal freight— which friends.

I didn't see them every day, even when I was still flying. We were scattered across all four points of the compass rose, from Alaska to the Puget Sound region. We each flew a hundred to two hundred missions a year, and the crew permutations could include any of about thirty flight-nurse partners and fifteen to twenty pilots. The majority of us fly out of three different bases. Our home worlds were often in completely different orbits.

But we'd spend twelve to twenty-four hours at a gulp with one another. When we weren't in the air, we worked together on the everyday grist that supports flying—safety in the aircraft and on the ground, clinical review and education, communication with referring hospitals and fire departments, equipment maintenance. The purchasing and restocking of supplies, the hiring, orientation, and recognition of staff. And when the day drew down toward dark, we watched movies and shared meals back at quarters while the wind howled down the runway and around the eaves, banged the drainpipe outside the living room.

And above all, we talked. People in our jobs tend to be humane and forthright, vivid and funny. Before you even realize you're forming friendships, you know whose child is a good student but hangs in the corner at recess, alone. You're part of a two-hour discussion on why your partner's son can't stay on task, whether it's normal or a sign of ADHD, and whether medication should be an option. You know whose marriage or relationship is troubled, and why. And you don't keep many secrets of your own.

Or at least, you see some stuffing that families aren't in a position to see. You sweat together through interesting times. Your warts show—your idiosyncrasies and irritations, the holes in your clinical experience and sometimes in your character. Your strengths show too.

Howie, knowing from the very fact of the call what the substance of it had to be, covered me with his warm fleece robe. I eyed my dresser, wanting socks. My feet felt too exposed.

"Police and Coast Guard are out there now," Tom was saying on the phone. They haven't found anything yet."

In your gut, the whole universe has shifted a degree or two, but your thoughts are on *where*. You think of the hour that has elapsed since they were last heard from, and your mind races up and down the terrain. There's hardly an undeveloped square inch between Seattle and Arlington; you wonder how a whole helicopter can disappear and nobody sees a thing. You know that the route back to base can run overland, usually east of the freeway, or over water just to the west of the shoreline, and that it's driven by conditions and pilot preference. Once a pod of whales decided the route. Ben, Tia, and I watched them surface and dive, surface and dive, from a thousand feet.

You also know it's the first gusty, stormy night of autumn, that tree limbs are crashing down in your own woods. Fog shrouds your deck, makes haloes of your outdoor lights, lingers under your trees. You know they had to be skirting some weather. You know the searchers are up against the weather too.

After you thank Tom and call Laura, who is scheduled to work in Arlington the following morning, you look over your husband's shoulder. He's on the Internet and has punched up a map of the Edmonds area. There's a large park in north Edmonds, dark and devoid of streets. You think it's nearly certain they crashed into the water. But you want to get out to that park with a flashlight and search for them yourself.

The National Transportation Safety Board, in cooperation with the Federal Aviation Administration, investigates and reports on aviation accidents. They have a Web site with a database, and reports are a couple of clicks away—our tax dollars at work. It is an efficient, user-friendly database, searchable by any of multiple parameters: incident date, location, severity, or investigation number; make, model, or registration number of each aircraft; type or name of operation. A table of incidents that meet your criteria is then displayed, with headings that show the details of each. Under the heading Incident Severity, the choices are *nonfatal* and *fatal*. *Fatal* appears in red, with the number of fatalities following in parentheses. When you click on a particular incident, you find a one-page synopsis and a link at the bottom: *Full narrative available.*

These are strange, compelling documents. The full narrative is formatted into sections. History of flight, plus a section each for personnel, aircraft, meteorological, wreckage/impact, and medical/pathological information, and a section for tests and research conducted. They're stories with beginnings, middles, and ends, the stuff of nightmares couched in a careful aviation argot, punctuated by startling quotes from witnesses. Aircraft parts sheared off in midair or upon impact, corroded by months underwater, or scattered across debris fields whose layout and dimensions tell a specific tale. Parts tested and found to have foreign paint on them from untoward collisions with other parts. Bodies that are found or not found. If found, tested for ethanol, drugs, and other toxins, and the cause of death almost always recorded as "blunt force injury."

There is a stack of these narratives on my desk, a stack whose stories mesh with mine in some fashion, head-on or at a tangent, to a greater or lesser extent. They average out to one for each year I was a flight nurse.

∞

#1

The year 1995, on what would become, six years in the future, an infamous date: September 11. Three and a half years before I became a flight nurse, two years before I relocated from San Francisco to the Seattle area. An aircraft and its crew crashed into Puget Sound one mile off the island that would eventually become my home. It was just before dawn, overcast—a cloud-cover "ceiling" that varied, in reports, from between two hundred and one thousand feet above the water. The ocean itself was calm, "glassy." At least three people saw the aircraft in flight; one on the Seattle side reported seeing it "fifty feet above ground level over Puget Sound. Watched with binoculars and saw anti-collision lights, strobes working and helicopter was straight and level, then it disappeared." There were several people who heard it as well. A typical auditory account from the island reported "heard the helicopter coming for two or three minutes. It was running perfectly at high RPM with no change whatsoever in RPM. Then there was a significant 'pop'—not an explosion—and then silence."

The bodies of the two flight nurses, Marna and Amy, were recovered in the debris field at the surface. The body of the pilot was never found. Most of the aircraft settled onto the sea bottom 750 feet below and was not recovered for many months. The probable cause of the accident, as determined by the National Transportation Safety Board, was that "the pilot failed to maintain sufficient altitude above the surface of the water, while flying over calm water conditions at night."

Of course I did not know the crew. But they were a presence all the same. An afternoon of my initial two-week classroom training was devoted to the crash and its effects on the organization, both practical and human. Their photographs and a memorial plaque hung in the main hallway of our office. An annual award had been established in their honor; I was a member of the committee that chose the recipient each year. There was a commemorative bonfire at a local beach each September 11. And once, when a colleague and I were updating the computer database of our equipment, we came across an entry for a defibrillator we couldn't identify.

"Which Lifepak Ten is that?" my friend puzzled, wrinkling

his nose. But then the shivery realization dawned on both of us: it was the one at the bottom of the sound.

Every day I flew with nurses who had flown with them, and their names popped up like corks in the eddies of conversation. Marna, I learned, had been calm and good-humored under duress. Once, a former partner of hers, who at the time of the storytelling was my partner, had dropped a laryngoscope handle during a hairy intubation; it had rolled away under the patient's stretcher into a dusty corner of the medic rig. Marna had retrieved it with a joke and a smile. When I heard their names and their stories, it was like hearing about close relatives who had died before I was born. The same dynamic. Marna, Amy, and Lee were ancestors, in a way.

#2

I was at work at our central base on a Sunday in late January 2002. I had begun to have vision problems in my left eye— a blind spot and blurring, accompanied by intermittent tremor, dizziness, disturbances in fine-motor coordination, and a constant, almost incapacitating fatigue—on Thanksgiving Day 2001. I was diagnosed with optic neuritis on December 4, and with MS on December 11. After a few unsettling weeks off on sick leave, I had returned to work on New Year's Eve, just twenty days before.

I was on F shift, which meant I was crew for our Learjet, used for long-range transports. I would be in house for twelve hours, on call for twelve hours. I wouldn't be free until 0700 on Monday.

On Saturday evening, a helicopter flight into the mountains had been aborted on the return leg because of worsening weather, including snow. They landed at the nearest safe spot, and the nurses and patient continued the transport by ground. Their pilot, Steve, overnighted at a fire station near their impromptu landing zone. On Sunday morning, with good weather restored and after a thorough preflight check, he took off just before 0800. Less than a minute later, at about three hundred feet of altitude, he lost power in one engine; he was circling around to land again when he lost power in the second engine. He managed somehow to avoid the nearby highway with its unsuspecting motorists and crashed instead into a small clearing in the midst of trees. The local firefighters who had secured his landing zone were on the scene almost immediately.

Medic response time was about one minute, and that, in concert with the skill of everyone involved in his care, might have made the difference, might have bought Steve precisely three years, eight months, and eight days more of life. The A shift helicopter crew, seated next to me in our workroom when we got the news, was dispatched to transport Steve to the trauma center. The reports started coming in by radio and phone. We heard he was short of breath at the scene but alert and oriented, with some fractures. That didn't sound too bad. Then we heard he needed to be intubated after a "buttload" of Versed, a sedative-hypnotic. Not so good. After he arrived at the trauma center, reports of his injuries started to mount up— injuries that could easily prove fatal, and that were concentrated on his left side, where the helicopter had landed. Lots of blood products, hours in the OR to repair delicate, vital structures. We took a little comfort from the knowledge that his brain was uninjured.

The left side of the aircraft was where I normally sat, and some nexus in my brain took note of the fact. I made calls activating the phone tree for the next hour. The phone tree was created so that sensitive information could be disseminated to staff members in an emergency without tying up all the phone lines. I had to force myself to dial the first name on each limb of it. To tell the news again and again.

Steve was slim, fit, in his fifties. Dark-haired, beginning to gray, a former military pilot with thousands of hours in the air. A quiet, dignified family man who was honestly devout and still in love with his wife after thirty or more years. I liked hearing about his dog, an improbable golden retriever/basset mix who swam in the waters near his home on Whidbey Island. People on shore would comment on what a beautiful retriever he was, right up until the moment he emerged from the water on his stubby little basset hound legs.

I flew with Steve fairly often, and he never failed to exude a kind of meticulous, courteous goodwill. On a transport, he always looked for extra ways to be helpful to my partner and me, and to the patient. He kept us apprised of everything he did at the controls of the aircraft. I felt *safe* in the air with him. And now I didn't know what would happen to him. A gory, detailed vision of his injuries was easy to conjure; I've seen them so often in others. The awful fact of them kept popping into consciousness as I made calls, checked aircraft, climbed into a helicopter myself to transport a sick pediatric patient.

The next day, there was the first of a series of debriefings. Ben, the youngest pilot in our program and one of the few without a military background, showed us slides of the crashed aircraft in situ and talked about what he'd found at the site. From our medical director, we received a graphic and complete update on Steve's condition, which was still grave. But information matters to people like us, and the details themselves gave us some traction on what had happened. Two CISM (Critical Incident Stress Management) experts talked about common reactions and what we could do to take care of ourselves. Ben led a prayer for Steve. Kleenex was passed around.

Afterward, a lot of us went over to the maintenance hangar

to take a look at the fuselage, which had been brought in from the crash site. There was a large hole in the skylight above the pilot's seat, and the floor under the pilot had caved in where it had landed on a big stump. The crew cabin didn't look as bad as I'd imagined it would, even on "my" side, the left side—I might have survived. It had been vertically compressed, however, and I thought of those forces transmitting through my spinal column and vital organs. My headrest was buckled, and my window was shattered. One of the pilots present pointed out that the main-rotor transmission wasn't sitting in our seats, so we wouldn't have been crushed to death. But Ben told me later that three of the four transmission supports had snapped, so there hadn't been much *keeping* it from sitting in our seats.

On Tuesday, two days after the crash, I worked a twenty-four-hour shift in Arlington with Ben. As soon as we arrived, at 9:00 a.m., we flew down to Seattle to attend another crash debriefing, less formal, more intimate. Thirty or forty people were there, and there was coffee and more Kleenex. Some were talking about their families—how their wives and husbands, their sons and daughters wanted to know they were safe at work, and how they couldn't provide that assurance.

I had discussed it myself with Howie, and with Kieran and Gabe. I showed them pictures of the damaged fuselage, all of us uncharacteristically quiet as we took it in. I shared every scrap of information with them. But one of the things I love about the men in my life is that when it comes to the Big Issues, they don't demand promises I'm unwilling to make or can't keep. They accepted the risk with me; they didn't ask me to quit. They never even hinted at it. And all I could tell them in return was that I didn't feel, in my bones, that I would die in a helicopter. As a rationale (or a rationalization) for a hazardous occupation, it's pitifully thin. But when I said that, Howie nodded. *Sometimes you get bit by the beast*, he said. *Steve got bit, that's all.*

It was an unusually vivid metaphor for Howie, weighted with metaphysical overtones, also unusual. And I think he meant that you can't see it coming, but also that the bite is random. You can't let the fear of it keep you from the business of your life.

Halfway through the meeting in Seattle, we were paged out. For what, I don't remember, except that winter weather again prevented us from flying all the way to our destination. We landed at the closest airport and waited for the referring hospital to ground our patient to us. My partner that day was from a distant base with a separate staff—I had seen her from time to time, but as a partner she was an unknown quantity. That might have been stressful, but I was tired enough not to care, tired enough to trust that we'd do fine together.

We talked about the potential causes of the crash. The theory seemed to be that a small amount of water or snow had been sucked in via the air intakes, snuffing first one and then the other engine. I heard that Steve had checked for snow in front of the intakes but that a small amount might have been hidden from view. And a helicopter can potentially land safely without engine power, by autorotation. During autorotation, the main rotor turns solely by the action of air moving up through the rotor, instead of by engine power driving the rotor. Since the tail rotor is driven by the main rotor transmission, it also can function without power. The pilot would retain some control over descent and heading. But since power loss occurred just after takeoff, at a low speed and altitude, autorotation in this case did not prevent a crash landing. I didn't understand every detail of the physics involved. But I felt in my gut the sluggishness of the aircraft just after takeoff, and it made intuitive sense.

Later that afternoon, we flew into the mountains for a scene response, landing behind a highway maintenance facility. We waited half an hour on the ground before the flight was canceled by the referring medics; we never even saw the patient. All three of us were relieved. On the way back to base, the mountains at our backs, skimming over the sodden fields of winter, we tried to sort out what we thought and felt.

Every member of the crew had the right to say, "I don't feel safe," and to refuse to fly or to abort the flight midmission. That said, there was a lot of weather where we operated and it varied in little microclimates all across the region. Weather was reported from fixed sites; it was not always possible to predict what we'd encounter at every moment during a hundred-mile flight. It was a fact of life, to be scud-running up in the helicopter, skirting areas of poor visibility in the effort to reach a patient.

Each person who flies, I think, has to evaluate the risk deep in his or her own core, and in his or her own way. I trusted our pilots, trusted their experience and competence. But alloyed with that trust was the knowledge that ours is a human business, necessarily conducted under suboptimal conditions for human beings. In weather, yes, but also at night and after long hours, when the vast majority of human bodies and brains press for sleep. The mean age for both helicopter pilots and nurses is rising—we're highly experienced but also prone to the physiologic erosions of time. And when most people go to work, they take off their coats in single locations, as familiar as their homes. When the three of us set off in a helicopter, the possible permutations of work environment were nearly infinite. Unpredictable, uncontrolled, unfamiliar. A systems nightmare.

Yet you adapt. You pan for familiarity, like gold. The helicopter becomes your home environment, and you know every piece of medical and survival equipment in it, and a bit about the avionics—the bit you might need to use in an emergency. You learn the quirks of each aircraft. You know which one's door handle sticks and which has a roof leak in a driving rainstorm. You know how to arrange things so they won't move or malfunction in flight, and how to keep track of them while loading or offloading. You're accustomed to noise, vibration, the radio and intercom, cold, heat, the buffeting caused by wind. You learn landmarks that help you orient yourself in the air. After several months of flying, you've been to all the usual haunts. One medic rig is much like another. You use the same landing zones over and over again, and you know where the landing-zone obstacles are, what they look like in daylight and at night. You know which hospitals have roof helipads and how to get to the ER and the ICU. You learn what emergency and health-care resources are available in each community; you meet the same providers again and again, and you can predict the level of care the patient received prior to your arrival.

But every situation has unique features, some visible, some unknowable. There are variables that no amount of forethought, planning, or systems engineering can control for. I think a realist accepts that dollop of uncertainty.

As we droned toward Arlington, I tried to convey some small shape of my thoughts to my companions. And I told them I didn't feel fear, or at least I wasn't aware of it as fear. What I felt was a decided lack of enthusiasm for the job, and it didn't center on the flying part, particularly. I didn't feel up to doing my *own* job, which was to provide the medical care. It was like a low-level emotional nausea—I could and did function through it, but since I'd heard the news on Sunday, I'd felt punky, under the weather. I think we all agreed on that feeling. And we talked a bit about our families' reactions. Ben was married to someone he loved too, and he had four young children; he had been flying throughout their lives. He moonlighted as a flight instructor, and he frequently flew with student pilots out of our airport before or after a shift with us. Later, when it seemed crucial to recall this conversation, I couldn't come up with any snag, any hint of unease or foreboding. We all seemed to have support at home for our careers; none of us mentioned pressure to quit. I told them what Howie had said about the beast.

"Yeah," Ben said. He sounded thoughtful. "That's right. He's right."

Ben was talkative, youthful, personable. He told me once that he thought of us flight nurses as sixty older sisters. He was also a devout Christian of a somewhat fundamentalist bent, on the opposite end of the religious spectrum from Howie and me, and the image of the beast may have had a different meaning to him. But in the aircraft, over the winter fields, we hadn't *felt* far apart. It had felt like we'd shared a moment of Zen.

A few weeks later, we (a different *we*, another of the many possible pilot-nurse combinations) stopped in after a flight to visit Steve. He was out of the ICU by then, on an acute-care floor, about to move to rehab. He was sleepy, perhaps a little sedated. But considering his life had nearly been extinguished just nineteen days before, he looked well. *Whole.* Amazingly, awesomely whole.

He told us that all the love and support he and his family had received in the wake of the crash showed him that we were his family too. He said he felt that God had been looking out for him. He said he didn't remember a thing about the accident, even though he had been awake and talking right afterward. He told us the latest prognosis gave him a chance for 100 percent recovery after more surgery and rehab, and that he intended to be back flying in five or six months. My partner told him to come back to us in September, after the brutal, trauma-season summer months were over.

I remember how grateful, how purely *happy* I was that he'd survived. How glad I was that he wasn't seared by flashbacks of the impact or its immediate aftermath. And to hear that he had a chance to return to real health—it felt as if I'd personally received a reprieve. It was an unexpected healing experience, to see and talk to him that morning. It brought up into the light of day a subconscious, visceral vein of unease and pain I had been harboring—and I wasn't even aware of its existence until I went into his room and held his hand.

More than a year later, the NTSB approved the following probable cause for the accident: "The sequential total loss of power in both engines 1 and 2 for undetermined reasons and the pilot's failure to maintain adequate rotor RPM to prevent a hard landing."

#3

Noon on the Saturday after Thanksgiving 2004. I had been on medical leave for a year, and another flight nurse had the misfortune to be on duty at our main office.

"I have to tell you that there was a helicopter crash this morning," she said. No good morning, no pleasantries. Her clipped New Zealand accent was particularly thick. My heart rate jumped, but before I could eke out a syllable she pushed on.

"It wasn't one of ours. But Ben was doing a training ride with a pilot who had just bought one of those little Robinsons— and he did not survive the crash. There were no survivors."

My ear heard the news, but it took a few seconds for ear to find brain, and brain to find mouth. "Ben . . . ," I said, and there was a silence.

"We're not activating the phone tree," she said. "Check your e-mail for updates. We'll get information out that way."

I'm not sure she even said good-bye.

One witness heard what he thought "was the engine making a loud noise, like a large diesel truck roaring, and then there was a large, loud bang north of my barn and some pieces fell to the ground." Several witnesses agreed the Robinson R22 Beta was at an altitude of three to five hundred feet just before it thrashed into the field. It "experienced an in-flight breakup followed by impact with the terrain during an uncontrolled descent near Arlington, Washington," in the stark language of the NTSB.

I heard that our crew—the pilot who'd relieved Ben that morning and two flight nurses—were put on standby to respond to the crash. They never left quarters; they were paged to stand down when it became obvious to the first-responders that there were no survivors at the scene.

Identification comes later. They could not have known it was Ben.

Ben took off with the student at about 9:20 a.m.; the nurses' shift at Arlington began at 9:00 a.m. Both the off-going and oncoming nurses might well have cheerfully waved to Ben as he went off to his appointment with the Robinson's student pilot. I had done it myself, often enough. And it's unsettling, to say the least, when I think of those black pagers with their klaxon of bad news, and the crew unaware of its nature. I myself would have been happy to hit the button after the page to stand down, happy to finish my coffee or complete the morning check of the helicopter.

The dynamic of cancellation was odd in itself. Flights could be canceled before takeoff or aborted en route by the requesting agency, and the reason was not always communicated. But the specter of death hovered around it, just out of sight. I remember one black, rainy wee-hour Saturday when I was on duty at our central base. "Forty-year-old male, head-on motor vehicle accident," our dispatcher had transmitted. The three of us, helmeted and plugged in to the radio system, tried to shake off the persistence of sleep as our pilot powered us up out on the ramp.

I tore a strip of two-inch-wide white tape and stuck it to my right thigh. At the top, I jotted an arrow pointing upward to signify takeoff and the time: 0204. It was the beginning of my documentation for the flight. We were just about to lift into the misty darkness when dispatch radioed again.

"Your flight is canceled. Stand down."

My emotional response to cancellation varied, depending on how much I had already flown, how exhausted I was, and how much energy I had managed to generate for the flight. Cancellation could inspire a newfound belief in the mercy of Jesus, augmented by the vision of warm blankets, or it could lead to a small sense of frustration because I was all jacked up with nowhere to go. At two o'clock in the morning, *Thank you, Jesus!* always prevailed.

It was possible our MVA was less injured than the first-responders had initially feared, and they'd found they could take him to the nearest hospital by ground. Ground transport is a lot cheaper for patient and insurer (if there is one), and it leaves air resources available for bigger emergencies.

But on the underside of that thought floated the words *head-on collision, 0200.* The Friday-night *bars* that had just closed a little while ago. The *remote area* the call came from. *Rain.* My partner and I exchanged glances and raised eyebrows. The aircraft felt a little hollow to me, like something small had seeped out into the night. It was my version of regret.

Back inside, I poked my head into the communications center, where our dispatcher sat in front of a bank of phone lines, radios, and recording equipment, twiddling a pencil.

"So, *is* he dead?" I asked, before I climbed the stairs to my bed.

A grim reaper of a smile played around his lips, and I knew the answer.

"He is no longer a taxpayer," our dispatcher affirmed.

∞

I can't tell you what a relief it was to return to a clean helicopter at three in the morning after what I could euphemistically term *a difficult flight*.

We actually called it *a thrash*.

A thrash could have any of an infinite number of causes— a cardiac patient developed a lethal rhythm, a trauma patient was bleeding out, or a child with meningococcemia lost her blood pressure as toxins from bacteria, exponentially multiplying, caused blood-vessel and end-organ damage. The common denominator of all thrashes was that a patient was trying, in some fashion, to die while we were in the air. Ordinarily, we did everything we could to anticipate bad juju before we took off, before we left a referring hospital's ER or the scene of an accident. We intubated and ventilated, we sedated and placated, we placed IVs and started antidysrhythmics or blood pressure medications. We took all the packed red blood cells available from the referring hospital. But when the shit hit the fan in spite of precautions, when the patient tanked as we were cruising over the mountains, my partner and I had no choice but to sweat our way through a full resuscitation in the tiny confines of the cabin. It was small enough that the bottom half of the stretcher, the part with the patient's legs on it, extended down into the cockpit to the space where a copilot might sit in some other kind of operation. We didn't have access to the entire patient, just the business end—head, thorax, and abdomen. Unless she was a pregnant woman in danger of delivering, in which case we loaded her headfirst, so *her* business end, her bottom, was where we could reach it.

The pilot sat with his back to us, on the right side of the cockpit next to the patient's feet, but over the roar of the engines and rotors, through our helmet headsets, he could hear us saying things like "Shit, his blood pressure is 60/20" followed by "I don't have a pulse, not even a carotid." The carotid pulse, in the neck, is the last to go. We'd urge him to fly faster, goddamn it, and we were only partially joking. We'd let him know we were out of our seat belts, rolling around like scattered marbles in the back, so he could steer gently. He would ask us periodically how it was going. "This sucks," we might both answer at once. Some pilots would throw in a quip or two for moral support. Meanwhile, my partner and I would thrust supplies at each other from our flight-suit pockets and the drawers under our seats. We would ransack the respiratory and medication bags, and there were never enough surfaces on which to place, say, a laryngoscope and a breathing tube until we were ready to use them. They would slide off onto the floor if we weren't careful.

Perhaps our primary suction would fail to respond because in my zeal to accomplish things in such a small space, I had kicked apart one of its connections. My partner would then have to dig out the portable unit. She would be grumbling aloud.

And there was often plenty to suction. Body fluids—blood but also vomit, mucus, and saliva (and on one memorable occasion, pink, frothy lung fluid from a young teenage boy in fulminant pulmonary edema from a methadone overdose) splashed around our tiny confines, spattering on the seats, on our flight suits and glasses. On the windows.

After a thrash, the cabin resembled the site of a depraved murder.

So by the time we rolled into the ER with one of us on the gurney, pumping on a chest; by the time we signed out at the receiving hospital on such a patient and spent an hour writing up the flight (having plenty to say); by the time we emerged from the thousand-watt fluorescence of the ER into the thin, existential moonlight of a January 0300, our adrenal glands had spurted themselves dry. My partner and I might have been eighteen hours into a twenty-four-hour shift, but as soon as we'd delivered the patient, we were officially in service and available for whatever mayhem would come next. We had to clean and restock ASAP. I learned to dread the endless hour ahead of us on the ramp back at quarters while we tracked and wiped away body substances from every surface, while we checked and replenished our gutted bags. Once the engines shut down, the only light sources were a portable camping lantern and the murky little beam of the penlight I held in my teeth.

A penlight which might itself have organic smears on it. I learned to clean it off first thing.

And we never got it all. In the blessed light of morning, the nurses who relieved us at 0900 would find what we'd missed— the perfect thumbprint of blood on the seat-belt buckle, the dried pool of vomit in the door pocket (if you reconstituted it, it would smell like beer). And if it was an exsanguinous sort of thrash, the helicopter mechanics would have to pull up the floor to clean under it, and not so much for aesthetics or even for infection control. Blood, it turns out, is corrosive to metal.

Aviation and medicine were separate systems in our operation, with separate job descriptions. But every one of the pilots would help us carry the patient from the field to the aircraft or lift him onto a gurney from the helicopter. It took four people to do it. Most would carry our medical bags when our hands were otherwise occupied. Some—Steve was one of them—would straighten up the back of the aircraft while we were in the ER after a *clean* flight. But they weren't required to know anything about our equipment or disinfection procedures, and a few, I suspect, were body-fluid phobic. That was fine. Their responsibility was the helicopter and flying it. Ours was the patient.

But while we were inside the receiving hospital, attempting to reconstruct the crazy quilt of the thrash on paper, outside on the helipad, *Ben* would clean the trashed cabin for us. He'd put on gloves and throw out all the bloodstained gauze and packaging that was knee-deep on the floor. He'd wipe down the monitor cords and the nondisposable probes with cleanser and disinfectant and coil them up nice and neat. He'd find the durable equipment and put it back in the bags. He'd scrub drying blood off the windows, track the stomach contents that had migrated from my purple nitrile glove to the door handle.

At three o'clock in the morning, after the gods of trauma had had their fun, the sight of a clean helicopter on the pad was a *gift* from Ben. It was nothing less than the chance to lay my bones down in a warm bed for a while, to sleep without dreams, like the dead. And our thrash patient, ventilated and compressed and transfused and shocked and slashed and lined and x-rayed, all to no avail, in the emergency department, had often joined that number. No longer a taxpayer.

There is little else to say, or else there is a world of things to say, too many. The new owner had bought, adapted, and installed nonstandard doors for the Robinson, but there was evidence that the door pins had *not* been installed. Both doors had separated from the aircraft in flight. The right door was recovered intact; the left door—the instructor's side, Ben's side—was in pieces. The NTSB found evidence of paint transfer from the tail boom to the left door handle, and to the leading edge of a piece of the main rotor blade. There was "a black impact strike mark . . . on the upper left side of the windscreen . . . consistent with a main rotor blade strike." Probable cause: "The divergence of the main rotor from its normal plane of rotation for an undetermined reason, resulting in rotor contact with the aircraft's left windscreen. The failure of the door pins to be installed was a factor."

There were no debriefings, because the crash was part of Ben's private life, not his employment with us. Our organization was not involved.

There was a very sad funeral. A huge crowd of mourners, many wearing flight suits. A slide montage of Ben's life—at the controls of several different aircraft, doing missionary work, playing with his children, constructing the new addition for his house. Near the end of the service, the arms of Ben's wife raised to heaven. And an obituary that was notable to me for one thing: Ben was exactly the same age as Kevin, my baby brother.

#4

Who's on it? I asked.

And Tom replied, and the hammer fell: *Erin, Lois, and Steve.*

I loved Erin, and I loved flying with Erin. She was a tall woman, one year older than me, thick and muscular with medium-brown hair and glasses. She had a deep, deliberate, deadpan voice—a contralto, as my mother would have pointed out had they ever met. Significant burn scars from a Molotov cocktail thrown at a high school graduation party, an injury that influenced her career choices. Like me, she struggled with her weight. We strategized a lot together about weight control; she favored Atkins. She was a good cook, and she brought real food to cook during a twenty-four-hour shift. She occasionally made me a yummy dish of baby bok choy when we worked together.

She was handy with tools, had a toolbox in her truck, and did many of the repair jobs at all three of the bases we worked at. She had recently bought land—and a rudimentary cabin she'd intended to remodel—on a river up north. The cabin had no plumbing or electricity, and she told all of us her drastic home-improvement stories. Some funny wiseass stuck a picture of an outhouse on the bathroom door in Arlington and penned in the caption "Erin's cabin." Even so, I used to wish she would come and remodel my house.

We had good chemistry in the air, in part because our skills —and our personalities—were complementary. I came from an ICU background and felt at home with the pathophysiology, level of detail, procedures, and equipment that came with that territory. Erin had been a paramedic for years before she became a nurse and then worked in hospital emergency departments prior to becoming a flight nurse, both with our organization and elsewhere. She was very comfortable out in the field. Hardly anything unsettled her, and many things amused her. She was outspoken and opinionated, and sometimes that bothered people, but I liked it. I think we felt safe with each other, confident that between us we could handle almost anything, but most of all we had *fun* together.

The tone was set on our very first flight, a fixed-wing flight for a sick adult ICU patient. I was brand-new, had been flying for perhaps two weeks. I was scared to death, in a constant state of stress that bordered on near-panic. The learning curve is very steep, and I didn't know if my progress was adequate or if I was considered a complete idiot. Erin was not my regular preceptor, but the flight was deemed a good learning experience, so off we went. I don't remember what the patient's problems were. GI bleeding, maybe. I do remember that she or he had arterial and central lines in place, and while Erin was taking report out at the nurses' station, I set them up so arterial and central venous waveforms and pressures would read out on our transport monitor. It was the easiest thing I had done in weeks; in my career to that date I had done it thousands of times, on many different monitors. And Erin was deliberate about taking report. She liked to be thorough; she didn't hurry as much as some others, and I had time. When she came back to the room, I had completely packaged the patient and we were ready to depart. It really wasn't much, but it was, like, the first time in the history of the universe that I had managed it in a timely fashion and with every detail accounted for.

Erin was not easily impressed, and yet she was visibly pleased as we rolled the patient away toward the ambulance that would take us to the airport. She said she didn't think she had done as well when she was new. The words were a lifeline. For the first time, I glimpsed a future as a flight nurse that encompassed *competence.*

Our joint karma as partners turned out to be busy, crowded with sick, sometimes unusual patients. A woman in her fifties with a thoracic aortic aneurysm, crying from chest pain, which made it likely that blood was dissecting through the layers of her aorta. Frightening because we were facing a forty-minute flight and it could burst at any time. If that happened, she would bleed out almost instantly.

A newborn from a tiny hospital with a congenital heart defect—transposition of the great vessels. In this defect, the aorta and pulmonary artery are in effect switched. Instead of deoxygenated blood flowing from the body, to the right side of the heart, to the lungs for oxygenation, then to the left side of the heart and back out to the body, blood flows in two separate circuits: oxygenated blood around and around the lungs, deoxygenated blood around and around the rest of the body. The baby was a slate blue.

A gray-haired employee at a rural bowling alley with a little alcohol onboard. He had wandered down to the end of the alley, bent down, and stuck his head under the pin setter, which had then triggered, pinning his chest just above the nipple line to the alley floor. He was unable to breathe for a time. When we saw him in the back of the medic rig, his head and upper chest were purple with congestion, and he was still drunk. We had to laugh about that one. He was lucky enough to recover fully.

One I wrote about in my journal, years ago. An unidentified young man in his twenties, also with alcohol onboard, had crashed his small 1980s pickup truck into a tree beside a secondary highway. After a silent ten-minute flight from quarters in the blackest part of the night—I felt shivery and exhausted, and Erin looked like I felt—we landed on the wrong side of the highway, deserted except for the pulsating lights of emergency vehicles. On our descent, we had seen the wreckage wrapped around the trunk of the tree; we could tell it had been a motor vehicle of some sort, but that was all. It was a heap of twisted metal and fiberglass. Erin and I stepped across the grassy divide through a cold swirl of fog and diesel fumes, both happy it wasn't raining sideways, and went up into the back of the rig. The medic had just intubated Mr. Doe, who was a large, rotund gentleman weighing at least three hundred pounds and probably a bit more.

Once we settled him in the helicopter, as we were lifting off, Erin stuck a flutter valve into John Doe's right upper chest. I pushed one in on the left and injected some morphine and a paralytic into his IV. I didn't want him to hurt, but I also didn't want his three-hundred-plus pounds to come up and kick around in the confines of the cabin. The starless dark streamed by around us at 160 knots, and we were aided by a tailwind, but we were still at least fifteen minutes out from the light and warmth of the trauma center. Erin popped IV #3 into a vein on Mr. Doe's upper right arm. She had the fluids wide open.

At 0300, when he'd hit the tree doing thirty-five, the guy took the steering column of the pickup to his chest. No seat belt, and no air bags, of course—the truck was too old for that. The nauseating sweet smell of semi-digested beer hung in the air around us. I threw a tube down into his stomach and attached suction; what was left of who-knows-how-many gurgled into a bucket at my feet. Mr. Doe, if he had been awake, would have said, "It was just a couple of beers." I'd love to have a dollar for every time I've heard those exact words.

Without imaging or other diagnostics, unavailable at the side of the road, we couldn't be sure what his injuries were exactly. But he had obvious fractured ribs on both sides, including the first two on the left. It takes exceptional force to break the first and second ribs. Blood in his lungs, a hit to his heart, large volumes of air and blood in the space around his lungs compressing his heart—all of these were possible. Likely.

Air had certainly dissected out from his lungs to where it doesn't belong. We could feel it popped up like bubble wrap under the skin of his chest, a condition known as subcutaneous emphysema. It was almost certain that air had also leaked internally, compressing one or both lungs—pneumothorax, the reason for the flutter valves. His oxygen saturation, measured by a probe on his finger, bore this out. After we placed the needles, it improved from the low 80s, very worrisome, to a near-normal 96 percent.

Our guy was awake and talking right after the accident, before the chest injuries led the medic to put a tube in his trachea and mechanically ventilate him. He wasn't making complete sense, so he'd probably taken a little hit to his head. Still, talking is high-level activity, a good sign for his brain, and the report of it cheered both Erin and me. He probably wouldn't be cabbage-patch material if we could just get him to the hospital.

The problem for us was that whenever we took our hands off the steel needles, Mr. Doe began circling the drain. His oxygenation and blood pressure both dropped through the floor. His heart rate fell. He tried to die.

My heart was pounding, but Erin looked thoughtful. She was as solid and unflustered as ever. "He's a big boy," she said, "and he has all this subcutaneous air in his chest. I think our flutter valves are a little too damn short."

I knew she was absolutely right. I mentally went over the contents of our bags. "Tough shit," I said. "There's nothing else we can use. We don't have anything longer."

We each pushed the needle in a little harder, and sure enough, oxygenation and blood pressure improved after a few seconds. Erin and I both grinned. I could feel relief, that rare liquor, seeping through my veins. I forgot all about nausea and exhaustion. We were wearing helmets and talking via radio over the thunder of the engines, but if it were possible to bend our ears down to the needles, we'd have heard the hiss of unwanted air escaping whenever we applied pressure. When the tips failed to reach their intended target, air reaccumulated around the lungs and collapsed them. It also compressed the big blood vessels leading into and out of the heart, so there was no blood flow and no blood pressure. It was a simple mechanical problem, basically.

It would have been a stupid shame for that kid, not much older than my sons, to die from a simple mechanical problem. Well, from drinking and driving, no seat belt, *and* a simple mechanical problem.

"Hey, whaling on these things works for me," I said to Erin, gesturing to the decent numbers on our monitor.

"Yeah!" she said, laughing. "How about that? Hands on, we're living the good life. Hands off, we're in deep, deep shit."

I eyeballed the drip chambers under the IV bags, made sure we still had plenty of fluid flowing into him. He was probably bleeding inside someplace. As long as we pushed those flutter valves into his chest, though, his blood pressure stayed up. He couldn't have been *gushing* from anywhere inside. We just had to keep him going another few minutes.

Our pilot set it down light and sweet on the hospital's rooftop. Erin held pressure on the flutter valves while I unplugged a bunch of things and got the patient and equipment ready to move. A couple of security guards helped us heave-ho the portly Mr. Doe and his backboard onto the hospital stretcher, and Erin and I wondered aloud for the hundred thousandth time how long our backs would last in the job.

I slung a bag over my shoulder and shoved what I had come to think of as "my" flutter valve into his chest with my left hand. Erin heaved our second bag over her shoulder and did the same with "her" flutter valve. I bagged breaths into him with my right hand, and we rolled him down the elevator and into the ER at 0355, just a little shy of an hour after he'd hit the tree in the middle of nowhere. His blood pressure was 134/75, his heart rate 105, and his oxygen saturations 95 percent. All pretty good, under the circumstances.

And the best thing was, it held up. So often it doesn't. Ten days later, when Erin and I worked together again, we called the hospital to find out that Mr. Doe, who was awake and had his real name back, was out of the ICU, sitting up, eating ice cream.

"Man," Erin said. She was leaning back in her chair, her arms folded, shaking her head. There was a sardonic little smile on her face. "I hope that guy isn't the scum of the earth. Because he was a *save*."

∞

In early 2003, Erin and I attended the same winter-survival training session in the Cascades. The entire day of training was predicated on a survivable crash (or "unscheduled landing") in the mountains. After a morning in the classroom, we practiced evacuation and orienteering techniques. We evaluated the optional survival gear we carried on our persons, which in my case was negligible. We practiced using the emergency supplies and equipment in the helicopter and learned some creative uses for pieces of the fuselage. We ate some MREs (meals ready to eat). We split up into groups of three that were each representative of a crew, and Erin and I were in the same group. Together with Joel and after several tries, we built a fire out of foraged sticks and constructed a snow cave together. A night in a snow cave, we all saw, would be a cramped, cold, viciously uncomfortable night.

And Erin and I joked about crashing. People did joke about it from time to time on the job, perhaps as a way to keep the bogeyman at bay, but at that session I specifically *recall* how we laughed about using the morphine and Valium in our pockets on each other for our injuries, as long as we had a hand between us that could pull it up in a syringe. In the backs of our minds, I think, were some of Steve's injuries. He was our model of a crash survivor.

And I wonder now (as I wonder about Ben, as I wonder about Lois and Steve) if she ever had an inkling of what was coming. Did she ever have uneasy dreams shadowed by wreckage? Did she ever, in the words of the old saying, feel a goose walking over her grave? She flew over the site of her own death several times a month, on average. But if she felt something, I never saw a sign of it. She, more than almost anyone else, loved the job. She was made for it. She told me more than once that she was constitutionally unsuited for any sort of normal nursing employment. A normal job, I could see, would have been way too confining for Erin. There would have been way too much compromising and too many fools to suffer. I actually wrote in my journal, more than a year before her death, that I thought she would die at eighty still in her flight suit and boots.

∽

I loved Lois too, but she was more elusive. Our friendship developed in fits and starts, spanned a decade and two cities. It honed itself as we bumped up against each other, again and again, almost by accident. Serendipity.

She was as different from Erin as you could imagine. Of Japanese descent, straight black hair. A chic short cut that never betrayed a hint of helmet head. Tiny, under five feet tall, but athletic and trim. Buff. Adjusted for scale, her biceps and thighs were huge, bulging with muscle. She was too short to fit in any of the standard sizes of flight suit, and she wasn't the type to swim in her clothes. She had them made.

We first met in San Francisco in the mid-1990s; 1996, I'd guess, though the years run together now like muddy streamlets. At that time, Lois was a traveler who took short-term assignments in pediatric intensive-care units all over the country, and I was a hospital-based pediatric critical-care float coming on to a night shift in a cardiac step-down unit

Nursing is a sisterhood. I suppose that sounds sexist, except that the many men in nursing are full members of it. And the quality of sisterhood is strongest among nurses in the same specialty—nurses who have done exactly the same work under largely the same conditions. There is so much commonality to draw on that friendships are easy to make and flare up strong, and they exist inside a time warp; if you meet up with a former colleague after ten years, you will usually be able to pick up right where you left off. Each specialty is a small universe. You can go to any PICU in the country, and as you talk to the staff, you'll discover a constellation of people you have in common. My friendship with Lois had its roots in the sisterhood.

For all that, I'm terrible at remembering names—they just don't imprint themselves in my brain—and I'm getting worse all the time. For years now, within the structure of our marriage it has been Howie's responsibility to match the names with the faces of people in public life: in politics, in movies, and on TV. If Howie's memory goes, we'll be a couple of clueless elders, adrift on the cultural sea. But he can't help me with people he doesn't know, people who are unique to my sphere, and my memory wasn't much better back in '96. At our first meeting, Lois introduced herself and reported off to me at 7:00 p.m. on our mutual patient. But by the following morning, when it was my turn to report to her, I had forgotten her name. I called her some other name, some wrong name, and she was annoyed.

"It's *Lois*," she hissed, gesturing to her name tag.

Years later, my friend and mentor Tia—who is Korean by birth and was adopted by a family from Idaho, where, as she puts it, "I was about the only Asian in the state, for chrissake"— informed me that if you're an Asian woman, a surprising number of white people assume your name is Susie or Kim.

"Like there are no other possible names for us," Tia said, laughing outright at the idiocy of it. And then I flashed on Lois pointing at her ID badge, her irritation a little out of proportion in my opinion for my transgression, and I have to admit, it might be true. I might have called her Susie. Or Kim.

But I remembered her name from then on, and she got over it. At that time, I lived four miles from work, a verdant, traffic-free four miles toward the sea, along the foggy paths of Golden Gate Park, and I ran home most days. It was a perfect distance for a workout and for mental decompression, and once I'd run the first mile it felt great. But inertia is hard to overcome, particularly when you've been up all night, and I sometimes whined as I changed into shorts and stuffed a few things in my fanny pack at the nurses' station. Lois egged me on every morning, one of those pleasant little social exchanges that you begin to rely on as part of the fabric of the day. But then her assignment was over, and she disappeared.

We surfaced together again in Seattle in another PICU, and

I was happy to meet up with her, a familiar face in a new city. Before long, a year ahead of me, she moved on to flight nursing, and I'd see her whenever she brought a patient to us. She encouraged me to apply to the flight program.

I never once flew with Lois. We were both pediatric flight nurses; we were not scheduled together as partners. But she was a source of support as I negotiated the learning curve. Her approach to the job was calm, considered, devoid of ego. After I'd joined the flight program, during the classroom training but before I ever set foot in an aircraft, she gave me a piece of advice.

"For the first two weeks," she said, laughing, "you'll be doing well if you can manage to buckle yourself in correctly. Just worry about that. Buckling your seat belt."

At the time I oriented to the job, the procedure was for a new flight nurse to go along for the first few shifts as a supernumerary observer. A regular crew was scheduled, and I was extra for a total of four flights, which were all that came our way on those particular shifts in early spring. It was the lull before summer, better known as trauma season. After those shifts, for the next three months, I was considered a trainee, but the crew on each flight was composed of my preceptor and me. It was like having one and a quarter brains in the aircraft. It was hardest on my two main preceptors, Brenda and Tia, who had to think on the fly of everything I might not know and who were forced to make up for my shortcomings. But of course the pressure was also on me to become a full, problem-solving, contributing partner as soon as I possibly could. On most of those early days, it felt like an impossible prospect.

Just buckle your seat belt became my wry internal mantra, shorthand for *Don't take yourself too seriously.* It provided that elusive thing, perspective. Sometimes I still hear an echo of that phrase when some species of shit is hitting the fan. I hear it in her voice, with her wacky laugh: kind of a loud bark at the onset then nasal bursts as it trailed off.

Lois was good at perspective, and she had a patient, dispassionate ear. When I voiced my early concern about my lack of emergency and trauma experience and how inadequate I felt at scene responses, she shrugged and said, "Yeah, well, you do ten traumas, you get the idea." It turned out to be true. I did ten prehospital traumas and got the idea.

Years passed. We worked on committees together, hung out in the office between flights. After I stopped running, she urged me on as a cyclist. We went out to dinner and the theater every few months. She lived in downtown Seattle, and whenever we went out, she picked me up at the downtown ferry dock in her little black Acura. She spent my July 22 birthday with me one year—we were almost the same age—and we went to Salty's in West Seattle by water taxi. Unaware that we were stranding ourselves, we watched the last boat of the evening depart as we drank our margaritas on the outside deck, our faces turned up to the long, late rays of our northern summer.

She had worked the day before our dinner date, and I asked her how her shift had gone.

"Oh, we had a barista flight," she said, deadpan, sipping at her drink.

It turned out Lois and her partner had been out in the middle of nowhere in a medic rig, stuck in Airway Hell. I've been there myself; I could imagine the scene.

You're in Airway Hell when your patient isn't breathing adequately, and none of you—none of the advanced-life-support providers on scene, nurses, or medics—can get him intubated. The list of potential reasons for failure are manifold. There might be facial or neck trauma with swelling or bleeding; the airway anatomy might have been disrupted. A heavy patient with lots of tissue in his airway can make it more difficult. A patient vomiting up the bowl of chili and the quart of beer he consumed an hour ago can gum up the works.

Once you've failed, though, your options are limited, and

you have to act quickly—with an apneic patient under normal circumstances, you have only a few minutes before brain damage begins to occur. You try to bag oxygen into him using a face mask—but it is suboptimal. It takes two hands and specialized positioning to open the airway and hold the mask to the face; you can't maintain it in transit. When you lose the seal, air leaks out around the mask, the chest fails to rise, your numbers plummet like meteors. You have sick sweat rings under your arms, your collective hair is sticking up on end, there's a tang of thwarted adrenaline in the close air of the ambulance.

Your next step might be a cricothyrotomy. This is a surgical procedure in which a breathing tube is placed through an incision in the patient's neck. Helicopters, medic rigs, and small planes are fairly "uncontrolled environments," as the vernacular goes, and you don't want to do surgery in them if there are any other options, particularly since you're not a surgeon. An operating room is on the other end of the spectrum. It is the epitome of a "controlled environment."

By virtue of its shelter and lights, bags of equipment and medications, suction and oxygen, the back of a rig or a helicopter *is* more controlled than blacktop or a muddy field, and sometimes your back is to the wall. In these venues, a cric is a slice-and-dice affair. A vertical incision with a scalpel under the Adam's apple; a helper to retract the edges of the incision and to sponge the wellspring of blood with four-by-four gauze squares; a horizontal incision into the trachea; a small hook to retract the edge of the tracheal incision while a tube is inserted. Then, with luck, eureka! Oxygenation and ventilation for the patient. For you, a flash flood of pure release as you see the chest rise with that first bagged breath, hear air moving into the lungs as your digitalized numbers improve from abysmal to livable. As you watch cold twilight seep out of your patient's face, a flush of dawn creep back in.

Nobody out in the field does this often. I've done it precisely twice, both times on an anesthetized pig in a lab, and animal-rights arguments aside (yes, I did feel bad about the pig), there are several orders of magnitude of difference between the pig and the pale neck of somebody's sixty-year-old mother glistening beneath your scalpel at 0200 on a moonless night, east of nowhere. But faced with somebody who isn't breathing, with a heart rate that's dropping and with brain cells dying by the millions, there's nothing left to lose.

I don't remember exactly what the outcome was for Lois's patient. I have a vague impression she or he did okay. But I stared at Lois over our drinks . . . *A barista flight?* I still didn't get it.

"Yeah," she said, and I heard a rueful version of the wacky laugh. "You know, the sort of flight where you think, *I wish the worst that could happen was to get somebody's low-fat-latte order wrong! Where you think: I wish I was a barista!*"

Lois loved the job, but she was clear-eyed about it too.

What would you change, if you could? It's the ghosts of our former selves I see when I think about Lois, brief blips of us outside patient rooms in the PICUs of two West Coast cities, in the front row of the balcony at the Paramount Theater, dressed in blue over countless cups of 0900 coffee at three different bases. On Salty's deck, that soft summer birthday evening. I miss her, and I want more than anything to reach back and warn her. But I can't.

Tia called me soon after Tom rang off. We compared notes about what we'd heard, but our information was minimal. It was nearly midnight by then, but neither of us could think of sleep. We decided to go to the main office where we'd be on site for any news. I would take the ferry over as a walk-on, and she would pick me up at the dock in Seattle. Howie drove me to the island terminal.

The boat was deserted on its last run of the night. I sat by the forward windows on the passenger deck and listened to the wind howl around pipes and railings. I could tell the storm was blowing itself out, but the ferry still pitched on the sound's chop, rocked by crosswinds. I cast an eye to the north, toward Edmonds, but saw nothing except night sky, roiled with low clouds. No moon.

The office was thronged with flight nurses and pilots, mechanics and dispatchers, administrators and friends. We learned they were last tracked over the water near Edmonds, and that weather, which had deteriorated right after they'd disappeared, had hampered the search.

The NTSB reports that radar data showed them "proceeding northbound over the water, following the coastline at an altitude of approximately 800 feet mean sea level. As the radar track reaches an area near Edmonds called Brown's Bay, the helicopter enters a left turn toward the west, away from the shoreline. The last radar return was recorded at 2112:33." They go on to say that no eyewitnesses were located but that nine earwitnesses on the Edmonds waterfront all reported the same thing. "Heard the helicopter fly by, then heard the impact. Called 911." The witnesses gave information about the weather. "Foggy in spots. Wind picking up from the west with sporadic rainfall. Mist. Conditions between drizzle and rain. Could not see the lights of Whidbey Island."

Soon after Tia and I arrived, the Coast Guard found a debris field on the surface of Brown's Bay, and not long after that, one body was recovered. Erin's.

We stayed the rest of the night. The mood was that of a wake. By morning, wreaths and bouquets would begin to arrive, scores of them, most of them from the fire departments, hospitals, and other agencies we served. As we all stood around in the halls throughout the wee hours, crying off and on, my boss told me that in the aftermath of the 1995 crash, she had come to hate the sight and smell of cut flowers.

"It was six *years*," she said, "before I could stand to have them in my house again."

In the days and weeks that followed, there were debriefings galore. Press conferences that I, thankfully, only had to observe, but that people I cared about had to conduct.

Some of the wreckage that had sunk 525 feet to the bottom was recovered by the navy in early October, and Steve's body was with it. The cause of death for both Erin and Steve was "blunt force injuries."

I remember how at a gathering after Ben's funeral the year before, Steve and I had talked about the weird experience of disability. How disorienting and dispiriting it is, in a way. My problems were invisible most of the time, and as we talked I felt like I had failed at something I cared about, though he certainly hadn't been aiming for me to feel that way. It was just that he looked fabulous, and he had moved heaven and earth to return to flying, whereas I was struggling with what sounded like the vapors of a Victorian maiden whenever I tried to describe it to people.

But it had taken Steve twenty months of rehab, not the five or six he had initially predicted. He had begun to fly again just a few weeks before I started my medical leave. As I drank my wine—I don't think he was drinking any—I told him I wanted to return too. I asked him how he was managing. If he was glad he'd come back.

"It feels good to be up there again," he said. "But I'm getting older. I think I'll fly a few more years—maybe two more years—and then I'll retire. By then I'll be ready."

At the time, I nodded. I understood Steve's wish to retire

on his own terms, not the terms that were thrust on him. But I think I also understood the note of fatigue in his voice. The degree of separation between what you want to do and what happens when you filter desire through your own resistant universe of blood and bone, of protoplasmic goo. There's a world of effort between the true north of intention and the magnetic north of achievement.

Again, that sense of time folding in on itself. What would I say now? If only.

According to the NTSB, examination of the recovered wreckage "revealed no evidence suggesting mechanical malfunction or failure. However, the majority of the helicopter, including most of the flight control system and all flight instruments and avionics, was not recovered, precluding determination of the reasons for the loss of control." Probable cause: "Loss of control for an undetermined reason during maneuvering flight, which resulted in an in-flight collision with the water."

Lois was never found. She's still out there somewhere in the deep.

There were memorial services, private and public. At the largest one, an honor guard of what seemed like hundreds of rigs from local and regional fire departments. At all of them, the ever-present slide shows of their lives. On the one hand, I was riveted by those brief living-color glimpses of my friends in times and places I'd known nothing about as well as in our own familiar haunts. On the other hand, it hurt to watch.

My own true moment of memorial was accidental. The morning after the crash, after we'd kept the vigil all night, Tia and I, along with a couple of others, volunteered to drive up to the

Arlington quarters to retrieve Erin's and Lois's things. I was relieved to have something practical to do, some way to contribute. I had missed everyone so much during my leave, much more than I had realized. I didn't want to go home yet, wasn't ready.

I knew the things they carried. Erin always brought a capacious, two-wheeled metal shopping cart to work with a messy jumble of things in it—tools and materials for those odd jobs she did, extra flight suits, paperwork for her committees, a T-shirt and sweatpants to sleep in, real food. Lois's style ran to one small duffel bag, zipped, so you didn't have a clue what was in it. It was never overstuffed, never straining at the zipper like mine always was.

And there was the problem of their cars. We intended to drive them back to Seattle if we could. Most crews left their keys on a table in the hangar so their cars could be moved if necessary. But not everybody, and not always. As Tia and I drove north to Arlington, we listened to a podcast of David Sedaris and managed to laugh. And we wondered if their keys were on the table or in some pockets of their flight suits. On their persons.

Sally had arrived before us, and she had collected their bags from the bedrooms upstairs. She handed me Lois's blue and white duffel. It had our logo on it.

The keys were on the table. Erin's burgundy pickup was next to an adjacent building, right where she usually parked it. Lois's little black Acura sat in a parking spot next to the hangar.

Erin was in the habit of smoking in her truck. Tia, who was an occasional smoker and didn't mind the smell, volunteered to drive it back to Seattle. Sally drove Tia's Volvo. I drew the keys to Lois's car.

Here's what I learned as I slipped behind the wheel: Lois

had been listening to the Mountain, 103.7 FM, when she'd pulled into the space at Arlington Municipal Airport and cut the ignition, twelve hours before she died. She must have liked the song that was playing, because the volume was *up*. She had just filled her tank; there was a receipt from the nearby gas station to prove it. Her car, like her person and her duffel, was neat, organized, and self-contained.

Since she was so short, I had to slide the seat back, something that almost never happens since I'm only five-three myself.

And I hated to do it. It felt all wrong, to begin to obliterate her presence that way. Because that's how it happens, really, doesn't it? That's how people fade from this life. Other people, living people, reach down and move the seat. I had been a passenger in her car many times, but it was freaky to wrap my hands around her steering wheel, blur some of her last fingerprints.

Freaky, but also a gift I didn't expect. An island of time alone with her, forty-five minutes of dodging trucks and cars, down through Marysville and Everett and Lynnwood and Shoreline. Through Edmonds. A trip she made so often, in the air and on the ground.

Forty-five minutes to try to *begin* to say good-bye. Maybe it was a gift I didn't deserve—there were so many others who loved her, family and friends. People more central to her life, day to day.

Nevertheless, the drive fell to me.

These days, my personal belief meter swings from agnostic to stone-cold atheist. But as I sat in her seat and swung her nimble little car in and out among the lanes of traffic thickening toward the city, my shoulders loosened and my foot got a little heavy. I kept the dial on the Mountain, and Sheryl Crow sang "Steve McQueen." I turned the volume *up*. For years I'd been driving a minivan, the plodding ox of the automotive world. Seventy-five in an Integra is a *whole* other thing. I opened up the window, and the cold salt breeze rushed in. It felt good on my cheeks. And in that subliminal stream of awareness that runs under the chatter of everyday life, I thought, *She doesn't mind that it's me making her last speed run down I-5.* I thought, *She's close by, isn't she.*

And the truth is, it felt like sacrament. Accidental sacrament, perhaps, but it's all I'll ever need, and as much as I can accept.

Acknowledgments

There are a legion of people behind this book.

Over the course of thirty years, more than four thousand patients and their loved ones have shared key moments of their lives with me—shared their most wrenching ultimate experiences. And minute by minute, as eleven thousand days have come and gone, each one of those patients has fundamentally changed me. They have allowed me to know beyond any doubt that human beings, however flawed, are amazingly resilient and courageous and good. I can't thank each one personally. I can't even thank the patients whose stories thread through this book, whose names are lost in the labyrinth of memory but who nevertheless seared me with their experiences, with their lives, and sometimes with their deaths. Whatever is best in me, I owe to them.

I owe another debt to my sisters and brothers in arms. To all those who are willing to roll up their sleeves and throw themselves into the difficult business of caring but especially to my fellow critical-care and flight nurses, who face extreme situations on a daily basis and manage, most of the time with flair and good humor, to create order out of chaos. Their resourcefulness and fortitude in the face of adversity, their intelligence, honesty, patience, and irreverence, have lit up my life for more than thirty years. There are no better friends on this earth.

As I worked on this book, I was continually buoyed by a rising tide of encouragement, generosity, and practical assistance. Much love and gratitude to my friend and mentor Judith Kitchen, who has been so instrumental to my development as a writer, and to Helene Atwan for her patience with me and her editing magic. Thanks and love to Kelli Russell Agodon, Annette Spaulding-Convy, and Nancy Canyon, who have been there since the beginning. Thanks to Gabe Culkin, an unexpected source of literary feedback and encouragement, and to the faculty, alumni, and students from the Rainier Writing Workshop at Pacific Lutheran University for their ongoing support. A special thanks to Robin Hemley for his guidance.

Material from this book has been published previously in slightly different forms. "A Hold on the Earth" appeared first in the *Georgia Review* as "Ichthyosis" and was later reprinted in *Utne Reader* under the title "Little Pea." "A Few Beats of Blackwing" appeared in the *Georgia Review* as "Asystole." Many thanks to Stephen Corey, editor in chief of the *Georgia Review*, for his kindness to a newcomer. A portion of "Omens" appeared under the title "Ghostwritten" in *The Jack Straw Writers Anthology 2006*. Thanks to J. T. Stewart, Moe Provencher, and the Jack Straw Foundation.

Thanks to Soapstone; Vermont Studio Center; the Washington Center for the Book; KUOW, Seattle's NPR affiliate; *A River and Sound Review*; Artist Trust; and the Rona Jaffe Foundation for residencies, resources, and funds.

And finally, thanks beyond measure to the whole tribe of my family, who have always loved and supported me.